Titles previously published in
YOUR PERSONAL HEALTH SERIES

Alzheimer's Disease

Arthritis

The Complete Breast Book

Crohn's Disease & Ulcerative Colitis

Cystic Fibrosis

Depression and Bipolar Disorders

Eating Disorders

Epilepsy and Seizures

Eyes

Hepatitis C

Migraine

Multiple Sclerosis

The Pain Relief Handbook

Parkinson's

Sleep

Stroke

When a Child Has Diabetes

YOUR PERSONAL HEALTH SERIES

ASSOCIATION MÉDICALE CANADIENNE — CANADIAN MEDICAL ASSOCIATION

Lupus

The Disease with a Thousand Faces

Edited by Dr. Sasha Bernatsky
and Dr. Jean-Luc Senécal

KEY PORTER BOOKS

Library and Archives Canada Cataloguing in Publication

Lupus / edited by Sasha Bernatsky ; with contributions from over 25 experts.

(Your personal health series)
Includes bibliographical references and index.
ISBN 1-55263-603-8

1. Systemic lupus erythematosus. I. Bernatsky, Sasha, 1967– II. Title. III. Series.

RC924.5.L85L86 2004 616.7'72 C2004-905361-2

The Canada Council for the Arts since 1957 | Le Conseil des Arts du Canada depuis 1957

Ontario Arts Council
Conseil des Arts de l'Ontario

The publisher gratefully acknowledges the support of the Canada Council for the Arts and the Ontario Arts Council for its publishing program. We acknowledge the support of the Government of Ontario through the Ontario Media Development Corporation's Ontario Book Initiative.

We acknowledge the financial support of the Government of Canada through the Book Publishing Industry Development Program (BPIDP) for our publishing activities.

Dr. Senécal is supported by operating grants from the Canadian Institutes of Health Research. Dr. Bernatsky was supported by a Canadian Institutes of Health Research/Lupus Canada Fellowship and is the recipient of a Canadian Arthritis Network Training Award.

This book is not a substitute for medical diagnosis, and you are advised always to consult your physician for specific information on personal health matters. The naming of any organization, product, resource or alternative therapy in this book does not imply endorsement by the CMA, the publisher, the editors or the authors; the omission of any such name does not imply disapproval by the CMA, the publisher, the editors or the authors. Neither the publisher, the editors, the authors nor the CMA assume any responsibility for liability arising from any error in or omission from the book, or from the use of any information contained in it.

Key Porter Books Limited
6 Adelaide Street East, 10th Floor
Toronto, Ontario
Canada M5C 1H6

www.keyporter.com

Diagrams: Theresa Sakno
Electronic formatting: Heidy Lawrance Associates

Printed and bound in Canada

04 05 06 07 08 09 6 5 4 3 2 1

To my wife, Nicole, and children Geneviève,
Isabelle and Pierre-Luc, for their loving support.

To my parents, Solange Dumas-Senécal and
Pierre-Michel Senécal, MD, who taught me to
strive for excellence and the importance to serve.

To Pat Leece, whose essential and understated role
in the first editions of Lupus: The Disease with a
Thousand Faces *prepared the way to this book.*

To our patients, whose dignity and fighting spirit
motivate us every day in the battle against lupus.

—Jean-Luc Senécal, MD

CANADIAN MEDICAL ASSOCIATION

This book is endorsed by the Canadian Medical Association. The association's mission is to serve and unite the physicians of Canada and be the national advocate, in partnership with the people of Canada, for the highest standards of health and healthcare.

Canadian Medical Association Advisor

Gunnar R. Kraag MD FRCPC
Professor of Medicine
University of Ottawa
Ottawa, ON

Contents

Foreword

You or a family member or friend have recently been diagnosed with systemic lupus erythematosus (SLE or "lupus"). This diagnosis probably is the result of a lengthy series of tests and procedures, all designed to either eliminate another potential problem or confirm the SLE diagnosis. It is not unusual for this process to take weeks or even months. Now you probably have a lot of questions.

SLE is a chronic disease with a variety of symptoms caused by inflammation in one or more parts of the body. It belongs to the family of diseases that includes rheumatoid arthritis, scleroderma and other conditions. SLE can target any of the body's tissues, and its manifestations are many. Because everyone's lupus experience is different, it's sometimes called "the disease with a thousand faces."

If you are having trouble absorbing all of this new information, you are not the only one. In North America alone, there are thousands of people affected with SLE. For example, some estimates of the prevalence of this disease suggest that SLE affected 500 people per million (close to 150,000 persons in the United States, or 16,000 in Canada) in 2004.

Like you, these women and men were probably confused and distressed by their diagnosis, and left wondering what to do next. Some plunged into research, digging up every possible piece of information on their disease; others felt more comfortable asking advice from a trusted family physician. What you decide to do and how you decide to proceed depends on you.

This book is a good starting point. Not only will it help you to understand SLE, but it will also play an integral role in teaching you how to live with the disease in a productive and meaningful way. You will find basic information on how SLE affects the body, and what you can do to manage and minimize symptoms, deal with various drug treatments, and handle concerns particular to women and children. You will encounter advice on coping strategies, and a resource section to guide you, should you wish to find more information.

SLE is, indeed, a challenging disease, but with careful management and medical assistance, there is every chance that you can look forward to a full and productive life.

"In the face of uncertainty, there is nothing wrong with hope."—Bernie Siegel, *Love, Medicine, and Miracles*.

Naomi F. Rothfield, MD
University of Connecticut School of Medicine

Acknowledgments

It has been our pleasure to serve as the general editors for this book. This publication grew out of an earlier patient booklet entitled "Lupus: The Disease with a Thousand Faces."

The Canadian Network for Improved Outcomes in Systemic Lupus (CaNIOS) is a group of researchers with a wide spectrum of expertise in lupus care and research. At our request, members of this network graciously agreed to work together to contribute to the new edition so that the previous booklet could be updated and expanded.

Lupus: The Disease with a Thousand Faces is perhaps the most comprehensive book on the subject written specifically for the lay reader. The expertise of the many contributors with whom we have worked ensures that the information presented here is both accurate and timely. Without their hard work and cooperation, this book would not have been possible. In order to properly acknowledge their hard work, we would like to list the co-authors here.

John Hanly, MD, Dalhousie University, provided information on nervous system involvement in SLE.

Suzanne Chartier, MD, Division of Dermatology, Centre Hospitalier de l'Université de Montréal, University of Montreal, contributed information on skin care in SLE.

Maryse Courteau, MD, Division of Nephrology, Centre Hospitalier de l'Université de Montréal, University of Montreal, provided information on lupus nephritis.

Tamara Grodzicky, MD, Division of Rheumatology, Centre Hospitalier de l'Université de Montréal, University of Montreal, provided information on the causes of SLE.

Yves Troyanov, MD, Hôpital du Sacre-Coeur, University of Montreal, and Jean-Richard Goulet, MD, Division of Rheumatology, Centre Hospitalier de l'Université de Montréal, University of Montreal, contributed information on antimalarial drugs.

Ann Clarke, MD, McGill University, provided information on the epidemiology of SLE.

Patricia Dobkin, Ph.D., and Deborah DaCosta, Ph.D., McGill University, contributed information on the challenges of coping with SLE.

Christian Pineau, MD, McGill University, provided information on antiphospholipid syndrome.

Douglas Smith, MD, University of Ottawa, provided information on the history of SLE.

Johnathan Adachi, MD, and Alexandra Papaionnou, MD, McMaster University, contributed information on how to prevent corticosteroid-induced osteoporosis.

Paul Fortin, MD, and Diane Ferland, RN, University of Toronto, contributed information on methotrexate, and on the CaNIOS research team.

Dafna Gladman, MD, and Murray Urowitz, MD, University of Toronto, contributed information on immunosuppressive drugs, and on morbidity and mortality.

Carl Laskin, MD, University of Toronto, contributed information on issues surrounding pregnancy and fertility.

Earl Silverman, MD, University of Toronto, provided information on pediatric SLE.

Steve Edworthy, MD, University of Calgary, contributed information on living with lupus.

Marvin J. Fritzler, MD, University of Calgary, contributed information on the ongoing research into SLE.

John Esdaile, MD, University of British Columbia, contributed information on the role of the patient and the doctor in the management of SLE, as well as on the use of prednisone in treatment.

We would also like to thank Lupus Canada for their support and encouragement.

Sasha Bernatsky, MD
Jean-Luc Senécal, MD

ONE

SLE: An Autoimmune Disease

In the foreword, you read that SLE (Systemic Lupus Erythematosis or "lupus") is often considered to belong to the family of diseases that includes rheumatoid arthritis, scleroderma and other conditions. What links these seemingly very different conditions is that, in each case, over-activity of the immune system leads to the inflammation and other changes that characterize each disease. Since SLE is a disease of the immune system, knowing a little about a normally functioning immune system is important to understanding what happens when things go wrong in SLE.

The Healthy Immune System

The immune system provides the body's own resistance to infection. The system is composed of white blood cells that serve specific functions (including some cells called T and B lymphocytes) and antibodies (made by the activation of these cells). The main role of the immune system is to protect you from foreign organisms that have invaded your body, such as

The Immune System

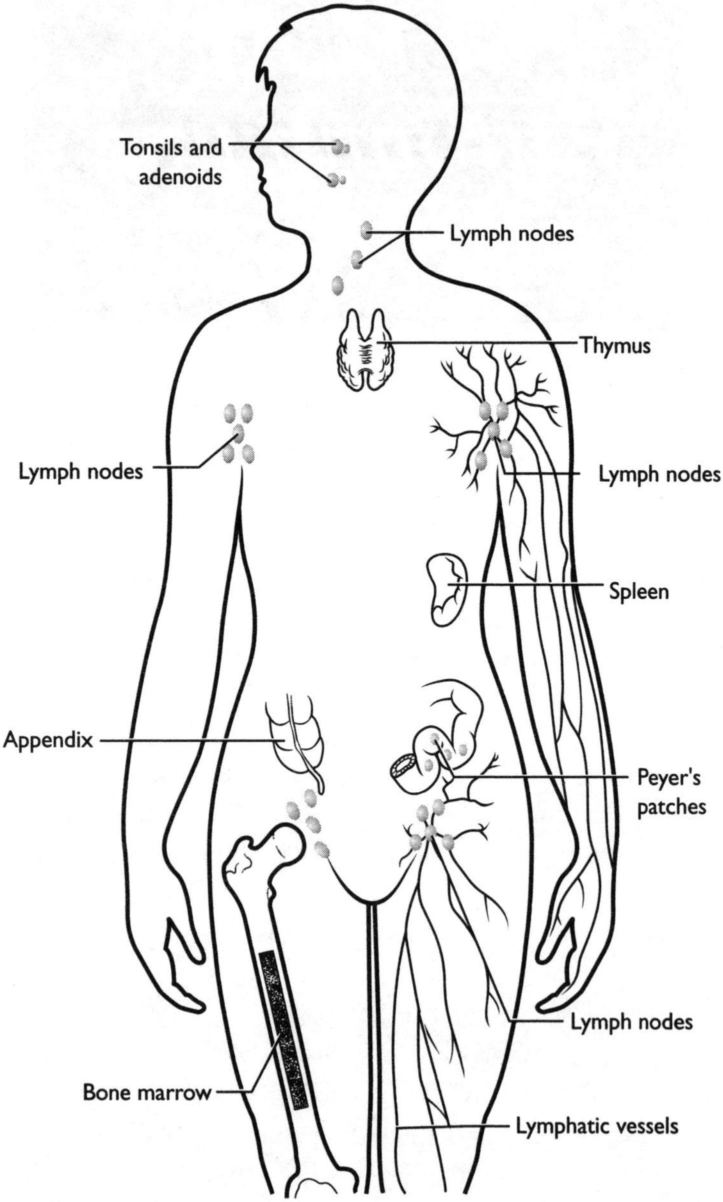

bacteria, viruses and parasites. When such organisms are present, the immune system is activated and attacks and eliminates them, thereby clearing infections efficiently.

White blood cells are made in the bone marrow. They form the body's patrol, on the alert for invaders. They also assemble in special tissue called lymph nodes. Lymph nodes and other tissues, such as the spleen, make up a sort of network of efficiently functioning lymphocytes. (See the diagram of the immune system on page 8.)

On activation, some B lymphocytes (see below) become a specific type of cell that produces antibodies—plasma cells. The antibodies produced by plasma cells normally target foreign (non-self) proteins called "antigens," present on invading bacteria, viruses and parasites. They are part of the way the immune system defends the body from infecting organisms. If instead the plasma cells produce antibodies against normal (self) tissues, autoimmune disease like SLE can result (see diagram on page 10).

B Lymphocytes

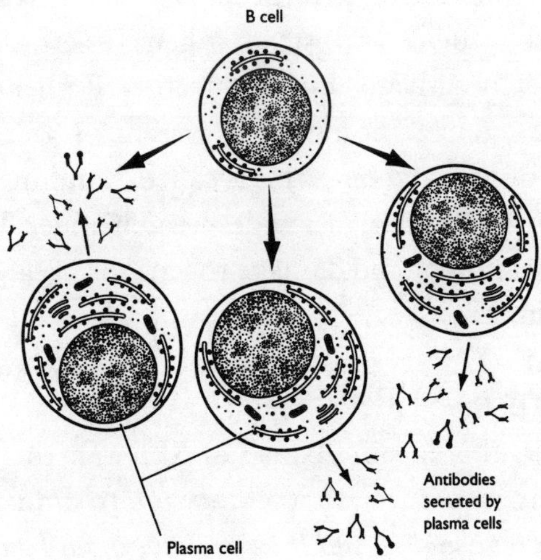

B lymphocytes can become plasma cells, which produce antibodies in both health and disease.

Antibody Production

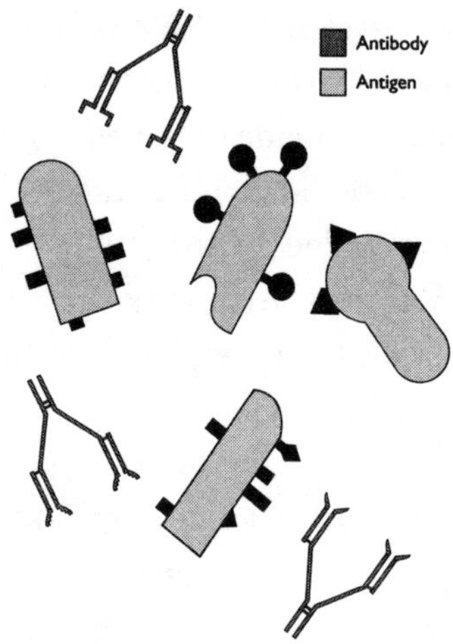

The antibodies produced by plasma cells are normally produced against foreign (non-self) proteins called "antigens" and represent a way the immune system defends the body from infecting organisms. If the plasma cells instead produce antibodies against normal (self) tissues, autoimmune disease like SLE can result.

The Immune System in SLE

In SLE, the immune system becomes over-activated and no longer works efficiently. Instead, it behaves erratically, and is inappropriately activated by many factors. Rather than attacking foreign agents, the immune system of an SLE patient attacks his or her *own cells* (this is called "autoimmunity," the term "auto" means self) in a widespread manner. This leads to the inflammation of and damage to various organs, the joints and the skin.

What Causes SLE?

To this day, the specific cause of SLE remains unknown. Although it is natural that you want to find the precise "trigger" or cause ("*Could it be the severe flu I suffered from last year?*" "*If only I hadn't gone south and spent my vaca-*

tion on the beach, I wouldn't have gotten SLE ..."), each factor taken individually is *not* sufficient to cause SLE. Rather, it is the presence of many factors—genetic, environmental, hormonal, immunologic and possibly others that are currently unknown—that determines *who* will develop SLE, and *when* and *how* the disease will occur and/or recur. They also determine the specific signs, symptoms and severity of the disease in any one individual.

Dysfunction of the Immune System

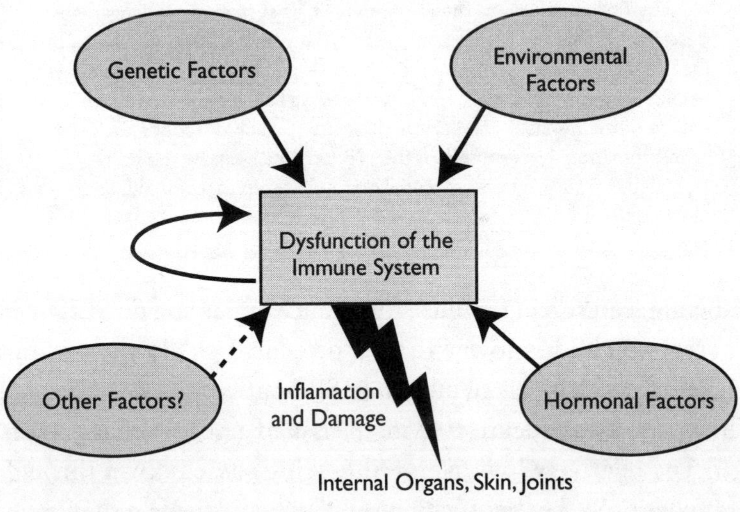

This diagram shows an overview of the many different factors causing SLE. The complex relationship among genetic, environmental, hormonal, immunologic and possibly other currently unknown factors leads to abnormal functioning of the immune system, resulting in the attack and destruction of one's own cells, with resulting inflammation of and damage to internal organs, skin and joints.

Is SLE Hereditary?

Genetic, or inherited, factors, are a part of the contributors to the onset of SLE. Although SLE and other autoimmune diseases (such as problems of the thyroid gland and autoimmune

We Have Come a Long Way

SLE is not a new disease. Hippocrates described a skin disease characterized by red rashes in 400 BC. The first known medical use of the word "lupus" was recorded in France c. AD 963. Between the thirteenth and sixteenth centuries, the word lupus was mostly applied to destructive ulcers on the legs. It was not until the sixteenth century that the use of the word was limited to rashes affecting the face. Throughout the eighteenth and nineteenth centuries, further clarifications, including an understanding of the importance of photosensitivity (that is, sensitivity to the sun) led to a better understanding of the disease.

Lupus as a systemic disease (that is, affecting the whole body) was first recognized in the late nineteenth century when two types of lupus were distinguished and a number of co-existing symptoms, including fever, nodules (swellings or growths), arthritis, swollen glands and pleurisy (inflammation of the membranes that surround the lungs) were described. The term "systemic lupus erythematosus" thus combines the idea of the potential involvement of the whole body, with two adjectives: "lupus" (lupus means wolf, and in some ways reflects the aggressive nature of the disease) and "erythematosus" (which describes the redness of inflammation, for example in the red facial rashes). By the early twentieth century, a detailed description of eleven cases of SLE had been published.

anemia) can run in families, the chance of passing on SLE from parent to child is lower than 5 percent. Usually the siblings (excluding identical twins) of an SLE patient are *not* affected; however, for an identical twin, the risk of getting SLE is greater.

The relatively low risk of SLE being passed down through families of SLE patients can be explained by the fact that many genes are involved: each gene contributes individually to the chance of developing SLE, but each is not enough on its own to induce the disease. This information is important. If you have SLE, it is unlikely that your child will develop it. On the other hand, if you do not have SLE, but your child does, do not blame yourself. Also remember that it is unlikely that a sibling will develop the disease. The genetics of SLE is an area of intense research, and much more information will undoubtedly be gained within the near future.

Are There Environmental Triggers?

The most important proven environmental trigger of SLE is ultraviolet (UV) light, such as direct sunlight and the light used in tanning salons. Ultraviolet light can induce chemical changes within skin cells that may activate the immune system. Although it is unclear whether exposure to UV light is sufficient to actually cause SLE, it is known that the onset of the disease after excessive sun exposure is not uncommon, and that flares of SLE often occur in certain patients after exposure to sunlight.

TWO

The Diagnosis of SLE

Who is at risk for developing the disease? How is it diagnosed? (Detailed descriptions on the symptoms of SLE are found in later chapters.)

Who Gets SLE?

SLE most commonly develops in women between the ages of fifteen and forty-five, although men, children and older people can also be affected. About eight times as many women as men with SLE are in the age-group fifteen to forty-five years. Overall, there are about five to six times as many women as men suffering from SLE. Although estrogen and other hormones may play a role in this female predominance, no clear roles have been established for them as a cause of SLE. African-American women are three times more likely to suffer from SLE than the general population, and women of Asian or Polynesian descent may have a more severe form of SLE.

How Is SLE Diagnosed?

Laboratory blood testing for SLE was first developed in 1906. Throughout the twentieth century, discoveries and procedures for testing have led to our present ability to accurately test for and determine the presence of SLE. Even with these advancements, SLE remains a difficult disease to diagnose. Because people with SLE go to their doctors with many symptoms that can imitate other diseases, the process of diagnosing SLE is often lengthy, taking weeks, months or sometimes years. For example, if the doctor suspects SLE but the evidence is not convincing, a period of careful observation may be necessary. Frequently, the family doctor will refer patients to a specialist such as a rheumatologist (a specialist in arthritis), an immunologist (a specialist in allergies and the immune system), a nephrologist (a specialist in kidney disease), a hematologist (a specialist in disorders of the blood cells) or a dermatologist (a specialist in skin disease) to provide advice regarding the diagnosis. If all of these specialists are not readily available in your community, further delays in diagnosis and/or treatment can occur.

The Lupus Team

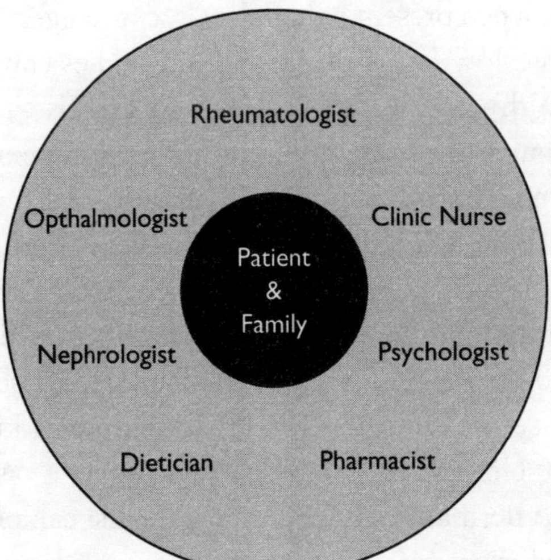

Your doctor will act on the advice of many healthcare professionals who could include the rheumatologist, the clinic nurse, the psychologist, the physiotherapist, the pharmacist, the dietician, as well as the patient and his or her family. Other specialists may be a part of the team providing advice, such as a nephrologist, if there is SLE kidney involvement, or an eye doctor (ophthalmologist) if the medication list includes antimalarial medications that warrant regular eye examinations.

When SLE is suspected on the basis of joint pain and swelling, a rash, etc., and/or blood-test findings, the doctor first reviews your symptoms, conducts a physical examination, and then orders various other tests, including the analysis of blood and urine samples, and perhaps X-rays. While some tests are targeted to specific symptoms (for example, a chest X-ray for shortness of breath), others are done to check blood-cell counts and kidney function, which can be affected without any outward signs. As well, testing for the presence of certain antibodies in the blood can help make the diagnosis. You may have heard of an antinuclear autoantibody (ANA) test. These autoantibodies, when present in high levels, can suggest SLE. However, because low levels of the autoantibodies can be present even in healthy people, the doctor must exercise great care in order to make the correct diagnosis. Consequently, further blood testing—for other autoantibodies that are more specific to SLE—is done, and if these autoantibodies are present in high levels, the diagnosis of SLE is more likely.

Other tests may be part of the search for a diagnosis. A biopsy involves the removal of a small piece of tissue from the organ that seems affected—usually the skin or a kidney.

- A skin biopsy can help diagnose whether a rash is due to SLE. A dermatologist or other specialist can perform this procedure.
- A kidney biopsy provides valuable information on the type, degree and age of SLE lesions and is often helpful

in choosing the right treatment. This surgical procedure is usually performed by a nephrologist or a radiologist (X-ray specialist).

Both procedures are usually done on an outpatient basis, although rarely a kidney biopsy might require a stay overnight in hospital.

Deana, thirty-one years old, felt that her energy had been poor for at least a year; and for some time the fatigue had been noticeably worse. Initially, her family doctor suspected thyroid problems, but subsequent blood tests showed that her thyroid hormone levels were normal. However, when she later complained of pain in the joints of her hands, her doctor noted that Deana was pale and had swollen joints, which might indicate arthritis. The result of a blood test to check her red blood cell (hemoglobin) level revealed that it was very low. Deana was sent to a hematologist who reviewed the blood work and suspected the presence of a "hemolytic anemia" that sometimes occurs in SLE. Further testing not only confirmed the hemolytic anemia, but also showed a positive ANA, along with other antibodies. The hematologist discussed these findings with Deana, her family doctor and a rheumatologist, who would be responsible for her treatment and follow-up visits. As well as having a new diagnosis—that of SLE—Deana now had a team (including her rheumatologist, her other specialists and her family doctor) who would work with her, with regular medical visits to monitor her medications and response to treatment.

As the case study of Deana illustrates, the diagnosis of SLE is never made on the basis of a single symptom or abnormal test—other abnormalities *must* be present. The American College of Rheumatology (ACR) has defined SLE as the presence of any combination of four out of eleven possible criteria. Although the original purpose of listing these criteria was to allow uniformity in research studies, in practice rheumatologists often use these criteria to make diagnoses. These criteria are:

1. Malar rash: fixed red rash over the cheeks (also known as the "butterfly" rash);
2. Discoid rash: red, raised, scaling patches anywhere on the body;
3. Photosensitivity: rash that develops after sun exposure;
4. Oral ulcers: sores in the mouth or nose, usually painless;
5. Arthritis: inflammation of the joints;
6. Serositis: inflammation of the lining around the lungs or the heart;
7. Renal Disorder: kidney involvement with blood cells or protein in the urine;
8. Neurologic Disorder: seizures or severe psychiatric problems;
9. Hematologic Disorder: low numbers of red cells, white cells or platelets in the blood;
10. Antinuclear Antibody (ANA): a laboratory test screening for autoantibodies. It can be present in many disorders, but suggests SLE if it is present in high levels and is associated with other SLE criteria; and
11. Immunologic Disorder: a positive laboratory test for various autoantibodies—one is the anti-DNA autoantibody test, which is more specific than the ANA.

Occasionally, an individual may have fewer than four of the above criteria, in which case and assuming that other symptoms consistent with SLE are present, a rheumatologist might make a "clinical" diagnosis of SLE.

SLE on the International Stage

In 1966, Edmund Dubois, in Los Angeles, published the first comprehensive medical textbook on SLE. In 1971, diagnostic criteria for SLE were established. These were further refined in 1982 by the American College of Rheumatology (ACR). The first international conference on SLE was held in Calgary, Alberta, in 1986. Since then, conferences have been held in Singapore, London, Jerusalem, Cancún, Barcelona and New York. In 1991, the first international scientific journal on SLE (appropriately titled *Lupus*) was published in London, England.

When you first receive the diagnosis of SLE, you will have many questions regarding what to expect from this disease. SLE is considered a "chronic" disease—that is, it can be mild or severe but will be around for a long time or the rest of your life. However, with treatment, SLE can be well controlled. You will experience periods of disease inactivity or remission that can last for months, years or indefinitely. The disease does have the potential to become active at any time, causing "flares" of symptoms. In this book, we may refer to these terms ("remission," "flare") as well as to "chronic phases" that may represent low-grade SLE activity.

Living with SLE

Survival in SLE has improved dramatically in the last few decades and continues to do so. In the 1950s, SLE was considered a fatal disease. Studies conducted during the past fifty years have shown that survival in SLE has improved significantly from the reported 50 percent survival at five years in 1955 to 80 percent survival at twenty years in 1995. The widespread use of corticosteroids and other treatments, better medical care, more timely diagnosis and closer follow-ups are all working to help patients with SLE live longer. The appropriate treatment of SLE, careful monitoring both of the disease and the complications of therapy and awareness of late complications, such as atherosclerosis, will help ensure you have the best possible quality of the rest of your life.

THREE

The Signs and Symptoms of SLE

People with SLE visit their doctors because of symptoms that involve a number of the body's systems. A symptom is an indication of something wrong that only the sick person perceives. A sign is an indication that someone else can see. Many times, more than one sign or symptom will be present during a period of disease activity. Often, the signs and symptoms of SLE that you experience initially are the signs and symptoms that you continue to experience. However, some people find that the initial signs and symptoms go away and new features develop.

In this chapter we will discuss how SLE can affect the kidneys, the nervous system, the clotting system and the skin. Other ways that SLE can affect the body are listed in Chapter Two (in the section under diagnostic criteria), and in Chapter Four (which contains a table giving examples of ways SLE can affect the body, along with what treatments are employed in these cases). These include the involvement of the joints in arthritis, the blood cells and the chest and heart linings.

SLE and the Kidneys

Normal Kidney Function

The kidneys are located in the back of the abdomen, on either side of the spine under the lower ribs. Shaped like kidney beans, they measure approximately 4 to 5 inches long and about 2 inches wide (12 x 7 x 3 cm) each, in the average adult. Their main role is to clean the blood of waste, namely the urea that is produced by the transformation of protein and creatinine (a chemical produced by the muscles). Kidneys act as high-performance filters: every 10 minutes, 20 percent of the blood flow passes through the renal arteries to the kidneys to be cleaned before returning to systemic circulation via the renal veins.

Each of our kidneys contains a million tiny filters called glomeruli. The glomeruli filter the blood and allow water, waste (urea, creatinine) and minerals (sodium, potassium,

Kidney Function

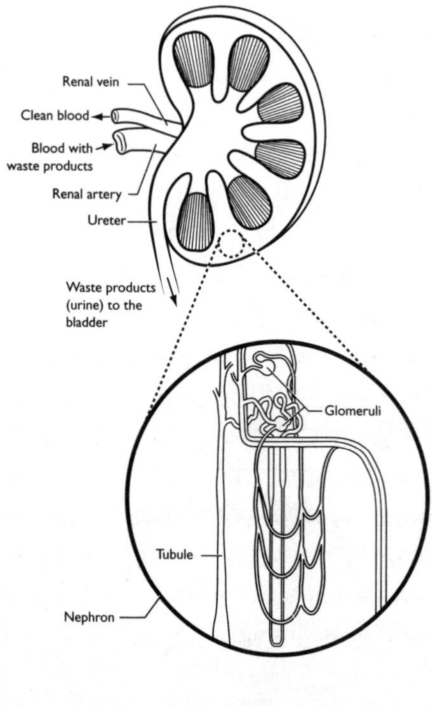

calcium and phosphorus) to pass through a network of tubes (or "tubules"). The tubules allow the return to the blood of the exact quantity of water and salt required to ensure the stability of body fluids. The remaining filtered fluid—containing waste—is eliminated as urine. Kidneys also produce hormones that regulate red blood cells and blood pressure. The urine is sent out to the ureters and from there to the bladder. Pierre's case study shows how a normal kidney works.

It's Saturday, and Pierre, a cycling enthusiast, completes a lengthy training session despite the summer heat. He is sweating profusely, to the extent that his eyebrows have become caked with salt. Upon returning to the gym, he weighs himself and notices that he has lost 2.2 pounds (1 kg) since the morning. He quenches his thirst with large glasses of lemonade and snacks on a bag of chips. His output of urine, which had been quite low throughout the day, gradually increases to normal levels. The next day, he discovers that the lost pounds are back. Thus, the kidneys adjust the quantity of urine produced on the basis of your state of hydration. Specifically, in the case of Pierre, the kidneys ensured that fluid was taken from the lemonade and salt from the chips to provide the necessary balance of water and salt retention in Pierre's body.

Kidney (Renal) Failure

When there is damage to the glomerulus, its filter membrane allows protein and blood cells to pass through (proteinuria, hematuria). If untreated, the membrane will react and stop its filtration process. Kidney failure will occur. The waste produced by the body's functions accumulates, and urea and creatinine levels increase in the blood. Kidney failure can be described in terms of extent (slight, moderate, severe) or length of time (acute or chronic). Someone with slight loss of kidney function might not have any symptoms at all. For example, we lose a little kidney function as we age, and older people can experience mild but stable kidney impairment that does not lead to complete kidney failure. On the other hand, many people with chronic kidney complications (as occurs in chronic diseases including not only SLE but also high blood pressure and diabetes) do have some progression of kidney failure, from mild (with no symptoms) to moderate (which may still be without symptoms) to severe (where fatigue, fluid retention, anemia and nausea become increasingly evident). Whether kidney failure progresses depends on many factors (such as the reasons for the failure and whether the processes are reversible).

People with SLE may experience kidney failure rapidly (acute) or gradually over many years (chronic). Since the symptoms generally appear slowly and often only in the later stages of kidney damage, many people are symptom free. Thus, people with SLE, especially those with known kidney problems, need regular kidney-function testing in order for their doctors to be aware of potential problems.

Inflammation of the Kidneys (SLE Glomerulonephritis, or Nephritis)

Inflammation of the kidneys is a potentially serious but usually treatable condition that is less frequent than other SLE-related problems, such as fatigue, joint pain or skin rashes. Approximately 50 percent of people with SLE initially have abnormalities in their urine analysis or suffer kidney failure over the years. This occurs more often at the onset of the disease or during a period when the SLE has flared.

Periodic testing is essential because there often is no outward sign of kidney damage. Your doctor will probably recommend you have these tests three or four times a year, even when the SLE appears to be inactive. These tests should also be ordered immediately if you feel the onset of any symptoms that suggest your illness is active.

Possible Signs of Kidney Dysfunction

Although kidney damage or dysfunction can often be present without symptoms, there occasionally are tell-tale signs. If you notice any of the following, you should notify your doctor immediately.

- swollen eyelids (often in the morning)
- swollen ankles (often at night)
- high blood pressure
- shortness of breath
- nausea and loss of appetite
- persistent extreme itchiness

Common screening tests include:

- a urine test (this should not be done during menstruation, as blood cells from the menstrual stream can contaminate the urine sample),
- a 24-hour urine collection to measure the creatinine clearance and the quantity of protein eliminated, and
- a blood test to measure creatinine levels, antibodies and complement levels (low levels of complement proteins may mean lupus is active).

Nina was diagnosed with SLE a year ago. At that time, a small amount of protein was present in her urine test. Dr. Osler, her rheumatologist, arranged for 24-hour urine collection and testing, the result of which confirmed his findings and showed that, despite the protein, Nina's kidneys were functioning at a normal rate. Dr. Osler believed Nina had a very mild form of SLE kidney involvement, and asked her to have urine tests repeated at regular intervals (including urinalyses at each clinic visit, with repeat 24-hour urine-collection tests depending on whether the urinalysis results seemed changed or stable). He explained that, in some kinds of SLE nephritis, decreased kidney functioning could cause changes, such as ankle swelling, shortness of breath and poor energy. He asked Nina to watch out for these signs.

The Kidney Biopsy

If test results indicate that your kidneys are affected, your rheumatologist may refer you to a nephrologist, who, after an evaluation, might suggest a kidney biopsy. This fifteen-minute procedure is performed following the application of a local anesthetic on the back below the ribs. Ultrasonic imaging allows the doctor to "see" the kidney through the skin and back tissues—and the sample kidney tissue is collected using a fine needle. The biopsy is done on only one kidney. Although the procedure does not take long to perform, it is followed by a few hours in bed to avoid bleeding problems. Analysis of the sample collected allows doctors to pinpoint the kind and amount of SLE-related inflammation in the kidney, and to establish the appropriate treatment.

The extent of kidney involvement in SLE can flare and diminish, just like all the symptoms of SLE. However, for many types of SLE kidney involvement, treatment with corticosteroids (prednisone, methylprednisolone) and with other medications (to be discussed later) is needed. Unfortunately, sometimes kidney failure or damage is not entirely reversible. Still, with careful medical attention—particularly with good blood pressure control—and attention to diet, good efforts can be made to limit the progress of kidney damage.

The Nervous System and SLE

The central nervous system consists of the brain and spinal cord. The peripheral nervous system is made up of the nerves in the arms and legs that control movement and provide sensation. The involvement of the nervous system in SLE remains a puzzle. The signs and symptoms vary from the commonplace (such as a headache) to the rare (such as psychosis). However, our knowledge of this complex and important area of SLE has been improved by recent advances in

- the definition of many of the different types of nervous system SLE,
- the development of new ways to evaluate the structure and function of the brain, and
- a better understanding of roles antibodies play in nervous system SLE.

The Central and Peripheral Nervous System

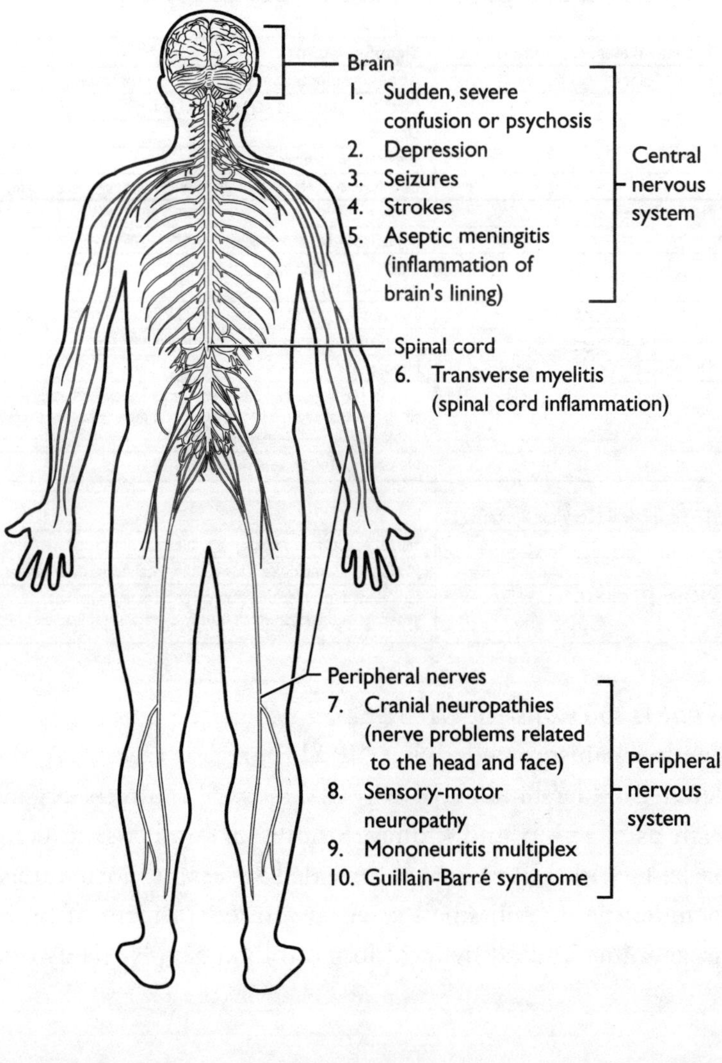

Classification of Nervous System SLE

More than 100 years ago it was recognized that SLE could attack the nervous system. Although a variety of terms have been used to describe this particular type of SLE, neuropsychiatric (NP) SLE is the best because it emphasizes both neurologic and psychiatric signs and symptoms, and central and peripheral nervous system involvement. Here is a list of the most common and serious signs and symptoms seen in NP-SLE.

Signs and Symptoms of Neuropsychiatric (NP) SLE

1. Central Nervous System	**Signs/Symptoms**
Diffuse (generalized) disease	Acute confusional state (sudden, severe confusion)
	Psychosis (Distorted perception of reality)
	Depression
	Generalized seizures
	Cognitive dysfunction (problems with memory and thought)
Focal disease	Strokes
	Focal (localized) seizures
	Cranial neuropathies (nerve problems related to the head and face)
	Transverse myelopathy (spinal cord inflammation or damage)
Movement disorders	Chorea (involuntary tremor or movement)
Miscellaneous	Headache
	Aseptic meningitis (severe headache and neck stiffness similar to that seen in bacterial or viral meningitis, but caused instead by SLE inflammation)
	Multiple sclerosis–like symptoms
2. Peripheral Nervous System	
	Sensory-motor neuropathy (symmetrical nerve involvement)
	Mononeuritis multiplex (non-symmetrical nerve involvement)
	Guillain-Barré Syndrome (rapidly progressing weakness, generally of the legs, which usually is gradually reversible)

What Is the Cause of NP-SLE?

The mechanisms underlying NP-SLE are less clear than the detailed understanding of why and how SLE affects organs such as the skin and kidney. Studies of brain tissue from patients with NP-SLE have revealed several abnormalities, including large and small cerebral infarcts (a form of brain tissue injury caused by local loss of blood supply) likely due to blockage of blood flow in medium and small blood vessels. These abnormalities may be associated with stroke-like symptoms (which can include changes in vision, speech, memory, power, sensation and other aspects of brain function), depending on the location of the changes. Infarct changes can be seen on imaging studies, such as CT (computerized tomography) or MRI (magnetic resonance imaging) scans. In people where such changes cannot be detected, it is thought that changes in brain cell function may have been the cause of NP-SLE.

Ongoing research is looking for the mechanisms of these injuries within the brain or other nervous tissue. Some intriguing possibilities have emerged over the years. Narrowing of small- and medium-sized blood vessels that causes a reduction of blood flow in affected areas may result from inflammation of the vessel wall (vasculitis) or more frequently as a result of the formation of blood clots within the vessel. Antiphospholipid antibodies, which occur in 30 to 40 percent of people with SLE, promote the formation of blood clots. These in turn may cause the stroke-like symptoms. Antiphospholipid antibodies are discussed in depth on pages 32–4 and 79). In general, abnormalities in blood flow tend to cause localized NP-SLE.

In contrast, diffuse NP-SLE has been linked to the presence of elevated levels of other autoantibodies (for example, antineuronal and antiribosomal P antibodies). These antibodies may be detected either in blood circulation or in the cerebrospinal fluid (CSF) that surrounds the brain and spinal cord. Normally, antibodies that circulate in the bloodstream are prevented from crossing into the CSF by an impenetrable structure called the blood-brain barrier. However, in some types of NP-SLE, this barrier may be damaged, thereby allowing autoantibodies to get into the brain. In other situations, antibodies may be produced "on site" by immune cells within the brain. As a consequence of one or both of these mechanisms, SLE autoantibodies gain direct access to the nervous system and cause damage to or malfunction of brain cells. In addition to the direct effects of SLE autoantibodies, brain cells produce inflammatory substances called cytokines; these molecules may also interfere with normal brain function. At this stage, it is unclear if the production of cytokines is linked with autoantibodies directed against brain cells.

How Is NP-SLE Diagnosed?

When considering a diagnosis of NP-SLE, your doctor will first exclude causes other than the direct effects of SLE. For example, complications due to SLE involvement of other organs, such as the kidneys, or complications of treatment, such as those rarely associated with the use of immunosuppressive drugs, can mimic NP-SLE. Therefore, a careful medical evaluation is the first step in this process. Then, there are a number of avenues to explore, such as:

- analysis of cerebrospinal fluid,
- assessment of brain structure (using an MRI machine), and
- a search for antiphospholipid antibodies in people with focal (localized) disease.

If you or your doctor are concerned because you are having difficulties with memory, cognitive function, concentration and intellect, a neuropsychologist can conduct formal neuropsychological testing to assess these important functions of the brain.

Current Guidelines for the Treatment of NP-SLE

Once a diagnosis of NP-SLE is confirmed, treatment will be tailored according to the individual's needs. The following principles can be applied in most cases:

- Identification and treatment of potential aggravating factors, such as high blood pressure, kidney failure and infection.

- Supportive and symptomatic therapy for specific NP problems, such as the use of anticonvulsant medications for seizure control and psychiatric medications for depression and psychosis.
- Therapies aimed at reducing the amounts or effects of SLE autoantibodies that may be causing the NP-SLE. For example, people with localized NP-SLE and antiphospholipid antibodies may have to take high doses of corticosteroids and immunosuppressive agents to lower autoantibody levels and reduce inflammation, and the use of anticoagulants (blood-thinners).

Treating Neuropsychiatric SLE

- **Identification of disorders that mimic NP-SLE**
  infection
  high blood pressure (hypertension)
  kidney (renal) failure
  electrolyte abnormalities (e.g., sodium, potassium)
- **Symptomatic and supportive therapy**
  anti-seizure drugs (anticonvulsants)
  drugs to stabilize abnormal and intrusive thought (psychotropics)
  medication for high blood pressure
  correction of electrolyte abnormalities
  treatment of infection
- **Immunosuppression**
  high-dose corticosteroids
  azathioprine
  cyclophosphamide
  mycophenolate mofetil
- **Anticoagulation**
  aspirin, heparin, coumadin

How Common Is NP-SLE and What Is the Prognosis?

Although NP involvement has been reported in up to 75 percent of cases, most recent studies have suggested that NP-SLE probably affects 20 to 30 percent of people with SLE. Research studies that have examined the prognosis for individuals following an NP-SLE event (such as those described in the table on page 28) have provided conflicting results. In some studies, there was an increased death rate associated with NP-SLE, while others reported no increase in the rate of death. Specific types of NP-SLE that occur with active SLE in other organs seem to worsen the prognosis. In contrast, headache and minor changes in memory, without other more severe NP-SLE signs or symptoms, do not seem to be associated with a poor prognosis or a greater chance of an early death.

Blood Clotting or Antiphospholipid Syndrome

Antiphospholipid syndrome is a condition caused by autoantibodies that lead to abnormal clotting. This syndrome can occur either as part of SLE or by itself in someone who doesn't have SLE.

Thrombotic Events

Blood clots normally form after an injury or a cut to stop bleeding. The abnormal formation of a blood clot is called a *thrombotic event*, during which a blood clot forms in a vein or an artery for no apparent reason. This leads to problems because the blood can no longer circulate normally in the affected blood vessel. An example of a thrombotic event is a *deep vein thrombosis*, where a blood clot forms in a large vein deep inside the leg. This leads to swelling of the leg that persists and is usually associated with pain and redness in the calf area. When that happens, there is a risk that the blood clot (or part of it) will dislodge itself from the leg and travel to the lungs. This is a

Antiphospholipid (Anticardiolipin) Autoantibodies and Thrombotic Events

The presence alone of these autoantibodies in someone who has never had a thrombotic event does not necessarily indicate a high risk of developing such a clot, since a large number of people have these antibodies and *never* develop abnormal clotting. Likely, there are specific characteristics of the antibodies (either related to binding ability or amount) or other predisposing factors that affect the likelihood of this happening. These characteristics are the subject of much research. People with lupus who have these autoantibodies should avoid those things that can increase the risk of blood clot formations, such as cigarette smoking and estrogen hormones.

potentially serious complication called a *pulmonary embolus*, which is associated with sudden and persistent shortness of breath, chest pain and sometimes the coughing up of blood. When a thrombotic event occurs in an artery, a heart attack or stroke can occur. If a thrombotic event occurs in the placenta during pregnancy, you could have a miscarriage.

Certain autoantibodies promote the abnormal formation of blood clots. These antibodies have different names, including *antiphospholipid antibodies*, *anticardiolipin antibodies* and *lupus anticoagulant* (which is a misnomer in that it is not actually an anticoagulant). They are all detected by specific blood tests. When these antibodies are found in a person who has had a thrombotic event, they are thought to play a role in abnormal clotting, and a diagnosis of antiphospholipid syndrome is made.

The Treatment of Thrombotic Events

People who have a thrombotic event are treated with medications that thin the blood, called anticoagulants. The main reason for this treatment is to prevent future thrombotic events. Common anticoagulants include medications such as heparin (injection form) and coumadin (trade name, Warfarin) (pill form). When you take coumadin, your doctor will adjust the dose after regular blood tests, known as the INR (for International Normalized Ratio) that check the degree of anticoagulation. Your doctor will decide how much medication is appropriate by assigning a range within which the INR should be kept. Anticoagulation medication is usually continued on a long-term basis.

SLE and the Skin

Skin problems are common in SLE. Listing all of them is not possible. However, three major forms of skin disease can occur in SLE. The terminology used to describe them is a bit confusing because, although these skin rashes also bear the name of "lupus," they may (like antiphospholipid syndrome) be present in the *absence* of SLE. The three forms are acute cutaneous lupus erythematosus (ACLE), subacute cutaneous lupus erythematosus (SCLE) and chronic cutaneous lupus erythematosus (CCLE). The pattern and severity of these lupus skin rashes can vary according to the severity of the underlying SLE activity.

Acute Cutaneous Lupus Erythematosus (ACLE)

Also known as the "butterfly" or "malar" rash, ACLE is a rash that occurs on both sides of the face (is symmetric) with redness (erythema) and swelling (edema) of the skin over the nose. The lines that run from the sides of your nose to the corners of your mouth are usually spared. However, the forehead, chin and neckline can be involved.

This type of rash can persist for weeks, and some people experience more prolonged periods of activity. It waxes and wanes with underlying SLE disease activity. Exposure to ultraviolet light is a frequent trigger factor for ACLE. The sources can be either natural (sunlight) or artificial (unshielded fluorescent lighting). This rash does not leave a scar and is rarely permanent.

Subacute Cutaneous SLE Erythematosus (SCLE)
These ring-shaped or disc-like red patches are usually *photosensitive*. In other words, they are triggered or worsened by sun exposure and therefore usually occur on any area that's been exposed to the sun. These rashes typically heal without scarring, but some pigment changes, such as whitening of the skin, can occur.

Chronic Cutaneous Lupus Erythematosus (CCLE)
Some people with CCLE have only skin involvement (a condition separate from SLE that is called cutaneous lupus, rather than the systemic condition—SLE). However, CCLE can also be a feature of SLE. The typical sign of CCLE is called discoid lupus erythematosus (DLE). *Discoid* refers to the appearance of red, raised, scaly and disc-like patches that often occur on the cheeks and nose. The upper back, the neckline and the back of the hands can also be affected. As they heal, these patches can leave white scars. Scarring on the scalp can cause areas of baldness that unfortunately may be irreversible.

Hair Loss and SLE

There are two types of hair loss in SLE; one is reversible, the other is not. Some people with SLE experience diffuse hair loss, mostly when the disease is active. This type of hair loss is usually short-lived and reversible. A dermatologist can help in differentiating hair loss due to SLE from other causes of hair loss, and make suggestions about medication that may help. The scarring type of hair loss is often patchy and associated with the discoid lesions of chronic cutaneous lupus erythematosus. These round patches may not always respond to treatment. Unfortunately, the loss of hair follicles due to scarring can result in patches of irreversible hair loss.

Vasculitic Rashes

Vasculitis refers to inflammation of blood vessels. In general this can affect any part of the body or body organs. When the vasculitis affects the skin, rashes appear as red or purple patches, often on the lower legs (although they can develop anywhere). The red or purple patches are in fact a manifestation of the inflammation of the blood vessels within the skin. In extreme case these lesions can develop into ulcers. Usually, vasculitis is treated with corticosteroids, and often with other immunosuppressive medications.

Protecting Your Skin

It is important to be careful regarding sun exposure, as indicated by the following case study:

For some time prior to her SLE diagnosis, Donna had noticed that her skin was very sensitive to sun exposure. She would break out in red patches on her arms after being outside. After listening to her doctor's advice, Donna is now very careful to

Taking Special Care

Skiers, climbers and all snow lovers, take care. Exposure to UV radiation increases with elevation, and reflection from snow and ice is intense. There are two kinds of UV rays—UVA and UVB. To be effective a sunblock should protect against both types of rays.

- Swimmers must take precautions because UV radiation penetrates water.
- Don't be fooled by overcast days: clouds filter less than 10 percent of UV light.
- Remember that wet fabrics lose significant sun-protective value. Stay in the shade beneath a big hat, an awning or a large umbrella.
- Remember that a significant amount of UV radiation can pass through window glass, in a building or a car.

avoid direct sun exposure, and always wears a hat with a wide brim and sunscreen of SPF (sun protective factor) 45. Now she can enjoy time outside without harm.

Clothing

Clothing is an excellent means of sun protection, especially if the garment is made from closely woven cloth.

- Cotton and polyester-cotton are both effective.
- Lycra may block UV radiation 100 percent when worn loosely, but it is less effective when stretched.
- Darker colors provide the most protection from the sun.

The most important factor for sun-protective clothing is the thickness of the weave. Some manufacturers market clothing lines with SPF ratings. In addition, special clothing designed for sun protection, such as Sunveil or Solumbra™, may be useful to patients. For further information, see the Resources section at the end of this book. To maximize sun protection, wear a hat with a large brim, and cover up with long sleeves, long trousers or skirt, socks and shoes.

Sunblock

Effective sunblocks have been available for many years, but their availability has greatly increased over the past decade. Although SLE patients should still avoid sun exposure, it is obviously impossible to do so completely. Sunblocks are a useful way to protect your skin from the harmful effects of the sun.

- Apply a sunscreen lightly to all uncovered skin before going outside.
- Choose a sunscreen with a very high protection; that is, one with an SPF of at least 30, or even 60, with ingredients that protect against both UVA and UVB.

- Look for sunscreens that have been endorsed or tested by a dermatological association.
- Apply sunscreen fifteen to thirty minutes before going outdoors, and reapply it every two hours or after exposure to water.
- Even sunscreens that promise all-day protection should be reapplied if rubbed off by clothing. Milky lotions are the easiest to apply.
- Alcohol-based lotions or gels are better for oily or hairy skin.
- Special sticks are useful for lips.
- Foundation makeup with sunscreen also offers UV protection.

Unfortunately, sunscreens can cause skin irritation or even an allergic reaction in some people. If simply changing the brand doesn't solve the problem, your dermatologist or family doctor can schedule patch tests to verify if you have an allergic reaction to a particular fragrance, chemical or preservative in the sunscreen.

Treating SLE Skin Disease

Often people who develop SLE skin disease also develop other types of internal organ involvement. In general, treatment is aimed at the most urgent type of involvement (for example, of the kidneys) and coexisting skin disease tends to get better as the other types of SLE are treated. On the other hand, cosmetic concerns are not trivial and patients with SLE should seek medical advice when the skin is the only area of SLE involvement.

Local Treatments

Many forms of SLE skin disease can be treated with corticosteroid creams applied to the affected skin until the rash has cleared up. Very powerful corticosteroid creams should only be used for a short period of time; a milder topical corticosteroid should be prescribed as the rash begins to respond to treatment. Ask the doctor who prescribes it how long it is safe to use a particular prescription. For more chronic or aggressive rashes, a small amount of corticosteroid medication can be injected directly into the affected skin.

Systemic Treatments

Antimalarial medications (for example, hydroxychloroquine, chloroquine) are very helpful in the treatment of SLE rashes because they are relatively non-toxic but often effective. Regular follow-ups are necessary. Occasionally, patients with severe SLE skin disease need treatment with corticosteroids given as pills (for example, prednisone) or, rarely, intravenously. There are more details on this treatment in Chapter Four.

Cosmetic Surgery

When you have severe SLE skin disease, you probably have been seeing a dermatologist (a skin doctor). If you are considering cosmetic correction for skin lesions that have produced permanent scars and/or color changes, consultation with your dermatologist should be the first step. It is sometimes difficult to gauge when cosmetic interventions can be helpful. For this reason, it is important to discuss any cosmetic treatment, including surgical procedures, with a dermatologist. If you don't have one, your rheumatologist or family doctor can refer you to one.

FOUR

Treatments, Drugs and Side Effects

At any given time, depending on the severity of your symptoms, the number of specialists who are involved in the management of your disease can vary. In Chapter Two, you were introduced to the potential members of your SLE team, which could include a family doctor, a rheumatologist, an immunologist, a nephrologist, a hematologist, a dermatologist, an ophthalmologist and others. The following discussion of roles applies to all members of your team. Of course, we are talking about an optimal situation in which all of these are available in your community. It may become necessary to travel to a nearby large center for consultation or treatment.

The Role of the Patient and Doctor

It is important that one of your physicians (often the rheumatologist) takes charge of your care and acts as the "SLE manager." Your family doctor, while not a specialist in SLE, will continue to play an important role in both your general health and the day-to-day management of your SLE. Family doctors are involved in the care of SLE patients for several reasons. Patients often live nearer to their family doctor or have other illnesses unrelated to SLE that do not require a visit to the rheumatologist. Family doctors will ensure that your screening and other preventative care—such as a cervical Pap test—be done regularly. They are also extremely useful in the management of problems that may occur in the course of treating SLE, such as high blood pressure or elevated cholesterol levels. The family doctor is also important because he or she plays an important role in supervising the disease when it is stable or in remission. Regular check-ups, usually scheduled every three months or so, will help this process. During these visits, the doctor will assess your general health and tolerance of medications. However, it's also important to remember that you too have a role to play in maintaining your health.

In SLE, as in any disease, patient involvement is crucial. Learning about SLE helps patients and their families be more aware of and alert to specific symptoms. Information can be found in books like this one, on reliable web sites (see Resources) and through support groups. An awareness of the signs and symptoms aids those with SLE to communicate well with their physicians. This can help the early detection and treatment of an SLE flare.

The specialist (often a rheumatologist) who oversees your care also plays a central role, of course. He or she will want to see you at least once or twice a year when the disease is in remission, more often when the disease is active.

Sharing Information

Effective management of SLE requires good communication. For example, letters, faxes and e-mail messages can be exchanged between the rheumatologist and any other specialists involved in SLE care and the family doctor so that all are kept up to date.

Mary is a thirty-year-old woman who has had SLE for ten years. When she was first diagnosed, Maxine's rheumatologist, Dr. Riviera, told her that Maxine herself would play a key role in the control of her disease. Through the years, Maxine has learned to watch for signs of SLE flare-ups. While initially she thought that her rheumatologist would be the only physician involved in her care, Maxine found out that Dr. Riviera appreciated the involvement of Maxine's family doctor, Dr. Munroe. Consequently, Maxine can consult Dr. Munroe both for non-SLE problems and for concerns regarding whether certain symptoms are related to SLE or something else. Both doctors stay in touch with each other so that each is aware of important developments, lab results and problems with or changes to medications.

Treatment for SLE is tailored to disease severity and specifically adapted to each patient. For those who may have mild SLE (that does not require any treatment), regular follow-ups with a physician are still necessary. Others with active SLE may need aggressive treatment and close monitoring. If you require treatment, your physician will continually reassess your SLE activity, adjusting your medications to minimize toxicity and maximize disease control. The stronger the treatment, the more frequent the reassessments should be. Remember that you are not alone in the struggle with SLE. As you work together, the goal of you and your team is always to monitor for problems and optimize your health.

Antimalarial Drugs

What Antimalarials Do

Antimalarial drugs, most commonly hydroxychloroquine, chloroquine and quinacrine, have been used in the treatment

Be Aware

It's important for people with SLE to be careful with their medications, since they are often taking complex combinations. Wear a Medic Alert bracelet and/or carry a card that identifies your medical conditions and the medications you're taking, particularly corticosteroids such as prednisone. Drugs containing sulfonamides (sulfa drugs) are best avoided because they can mimic an SLE flare by causing fever, arthritis, skin rashes, sun sensitivity and other problems. These drugs include some antibiotics, such as trimethoprim-sulfamethoxazole, that are used in the treatment of bladder or respiratory infections.

Before taking any new medication or alternative medicine (including over-the-counter drugs) always discuss your SLE and what you are currently taking with your doctor or pharmacist. New treatments can interact with your existing medications.

of SLE since the 1950s. They are called *antimalarials* because they were originally used against malaria, an infectious disease that is common outside North America and Europe. During World War II, soldiers took antimalarial drugs to prevent malaria. Stories among British troops of improvement of some skin diseases led to the drugs being used for patients with SLE and rheumatoid arthritis. It is not exactly known why antimalarials have beneficial effects on the immune system, but they appear to neutralize the autoimmunity that underlies problems such as SLE and related diseases.

The beneficial effects of antimalarials are not seen right away—these are slow-acting drugs. It may take up to six months, and sometimes longer, for the beneficial effects of this type of drug to be fully appreciated. Beneficial effects on rashes can nevertheless be seen in as early as a few weeks.

The effectiveness and low toxicity of antimalarial drugs have resulted in their extensive use for treating SLE. Nowadays many people with SLE will take an antimalarial for extended periods, such as ten years or more. To decrease the exposure to the drug, your doctor may adjust doses so that the lowest possible effective dose will be used. For example, doctors may administer the drug only during the summer months to people for whom photosensitive skin rashes are the primary indication for treatment.

Benefits

The antimalarials are often very effective in treating several of the numerous skin manifestations of SLE. They can be helpful against hair loss, ulcers of the nose and mouth, the malar or "butterfly" rash and hives, for example. The antimalarials can also be useful for relieving arthritis, fatigue and serositis (that is, inflammation of the lung [pleuritis] or heart [pericarditis] linings, which is associated with pain).

These drugs help to prevent flares of SLE. This was confirmed by Canadian rheumatologists in a study that was published in the *New England Journal of Medicine* in 1991. When hydroxychloroquine was withdrawn from people with inactive SLE, their SLE worsened compared with people who continued that medication. This study has encouraged long-term treatment with this agent. It is now widely believed that the use of antimalarials diminishes the overall need for corticosteroids such as prednisone.

Antimalarials also appear to counteract risk factors for heart disease. Premature heart disease is common in SLE patients. The many contributing factors include use of corticosteroids; the traditional risk factors of high blood pressure, diabetes, smoking and high cholesterol; and even SLE itself. Antimalarial drugs may prevent the increase in cholesterol seen in patients receiving steroid therapy. Hydroxychloroquine may even lower blood sugar in diabetic patients. The effect of antimalarials in decreasing SLE activity may also help in preventing premature heart disease. (Note, however, that antimalarials are *not* a substitute for other preventive measures, such as exercising and not smoking.)

Studies suggest that antimalarials decrease the risk of blood clots and strokes in people with antiphospholipid antibodies. However, antimalarial drugs are not a substitute for blood thinners (anticoagulants) for people who already have clots or strokes.

Side Effects

Antimalarial drugs are probably the safest anti-SLE drugs in use. To varying degrees, most immunosuppressive drugs used in SLE increase the risk of infections; antimalarials do not. Also, most rheumatologists now believe that hydroxychloroquine can be safely used in pregnancy. This is because, unlike many anti-SLE drugs, such as methotrexate or cyclophosphamide, antimalarials are not associated with high risk of harm to the baby. Since one of the major factors determining pregnancy outcome in SLE patients is the activity of SLE, and since discontinuing antimalarials can lead to flares (which can harm both the mother and the unborn child), many doctors feel that it is safer to continue hydroxychloroquine rather than to discontinue this drug simply because of pregnancy. Some rheumatologists are not as comfortable using this drug in pregnancy. (More information on the use of hydroxychloroquine in pregnancy and also in breastfeeding is available in Chapter Six.)

Short-term Effects

Minor but unpleasant side effects can sometimes be experienced in the first few weeks of treatment. Loose stools, diarrhea, abdominal cramps and nausea are not uncommon. These symptoms tend to decrease after a few weeks of treatment, or may require a reduction in the dose.

Long-term Effects

The most serious possible complication of chloroquine and hydroxychloroquine is damage to the eyes, specifically to the retina, the lining of the back of the eye, that can interfere with vision. Permanent loss of vision has only occurred in a very small number of patients taking antimalarials. However, all patients taking antimalarial drugs should have yearly or more frequent visits to an eye doctor (ophthalmologist), who can check you periodically for early problems, with careful, thorough examination of the eyes. Some ophthalmologists will give patients a self-monitoring tool called an Amsler grid, which is a sheet of paper with a grid of lines (see page 47). You can examine the Amsler grid between eye doctor visits. To administer the test, hold the Amsler Grid at eye level at a comfortable level. (If you wear any type of reading lenses, make sure you have them on.) Cover one eye at a time and focus on the center dot. If you notice a change in vision, such as faded squares, you should report it immediately to your doctor and have your vision checked. If the doctor detects early signs of retinal damage, the antimalarial drug will be stopped immediately to prevent more severe problems.

Eye damage related to antimalarial agents is rare and is largely dependent on dose. The risk of damage is very low if the daily dose of hydroxychloroquine is kept to no more than 6.5 mg/kg (based on your ideal body weight) although lower amounts should be used if you have kidney or liver damage. This approach, along with regular visits to the ophthalmologist, will make significant retinal damage an extremely uncommon side effect.

Even if you feel well but are taking antimalarial medications, it is very important that you visit the ophthalmologist regularly. You should have eye exams yearly within the first few years of beginning the medication, and twice a year (or more often) thereafter.

Amsler Grid

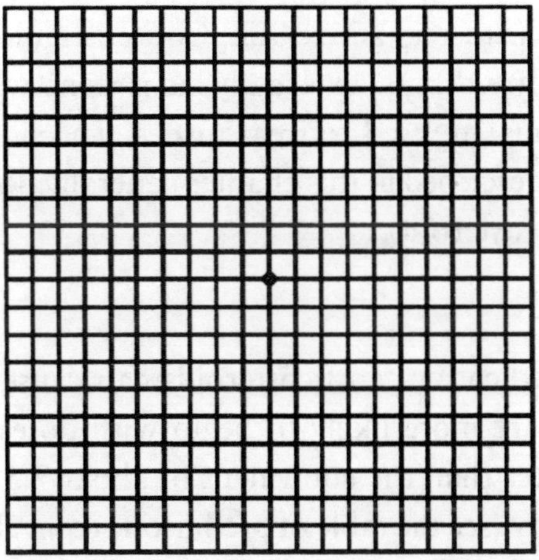

As a final note, antimalarials work best for people who do not smoke. This is another good reason for people with SLE to not smoke!

Corticosteroids

The discovery of corticosteroid drugs, such as prednisone, methylprednisolone and prednisolone, has led to quite an increase in the life expectancy of people with SLE. Corticosteroids are extremely effective in controlling SLE symptoms. But, like any other medication, they can cause side effects, some of which are quite serious. Generally, the goal is to taper the dosage of these drugs off to the minimum dose that allows for disease control. Most short-term side effects are reversible and, if necessary, treatable. Preventive measures significantly decrease the effect of several long-term side effects of corticosteroids.

What Corticosteroids Do

Corticosteroids are prescribed to quickly improve uncontrolled disease in SLE, especially if it is severe or life threatening. Some forms of corticosteroids (for example, prednisone) are taken orally as pills; others are given intravenously (by injection). This is done with very active SLE. Corticosteroids can also be used topically—that is, externally, as is done when corticosteroids creams are used to treat rashes. The side effects and monitoring described in this chapter generally do not apply to topical corticosteroids.

Side Effects

Like any medication, corticosteroids can cause side effects. Side effects are more likely to begin with doses of corticosteroids greater than the equivalent of about 7.5 mg of prednisone per day (see the table of prednisone equivalents on page 149). The higher the dose and the more prolonged the treatment, the more likely it is that side effects will occur. Conversely, the lower the dose and the shorter the treatment, the less likely are side effects. It is important to be aware that even at high doses, not everyone will develop all the effects listed. Unfortunately, it is not possible to detach corticosteroids' beneficial effects on SLE from their side effects. However unpleasant, the side effects do indicate that corticosteroids are being picked up by the body to act against SLE. Also, most of the short-term side effects are reversible: they go away when the dose is decreased.

Short-term Side Effects

1. Facial changes and weight gain: Corticosteroids often greatly increase appetite, which can lead to weight gain. Be persistent with your diet and, if possible, maintain an exercise regimen. High doses of corticosteroids can also lead to a redistribution of fat cells to the face and upper part of the back. These changes can be distressing, but remember that they indicate that the drug is working and keep in mind that these changes are reversible.

Getting It Right

How doctors determine both appropriate dosages and when to alter them depends on many factors. For example, while it is possible to decrease a dose primarily to get rid of adverse effects, the need to limit side effects must be balanced against the risk of not adequately controlling SLE activity. Often, other drugs are prescribed in addition to corticosteroids to control SLE, but these generally take longer to work. Thus, you may have to tolerate some unwanted effects of corticosteroids for the period (usually several weeks, or even several months) that it takes for the other drugs to take effect.

2. Mood: Some people find their mood and energy improves while others complain of depression, irritability or difficulty sleeping. After first discussing with your doctor, try taking the corticosteroids earlier in the day, which might help with the sleep problems. When the dose is decreased, most people find these problems resolve themselves.
3. Acne: Some patients get acne.
4. Facial hair: Occasionally some people notice changes in facial hair (it may become a bit coarser or more plentiful).
5. Upset stomach: This is often improved if you take corticosteroids with food. Your doctor might also prescribe a medication to relieve your symptoms. Stomach pain that is severe or associated with vomiting requires you to consult your doctor.
6. High blood sugar (hyperglycemia): Corticosteroids tend to cause higher than normal blood sugar (glucose) levels. If you are a diabetic, you may require changes in your diabetes therapy. Even if you are not a diabetic, corticosteroids can reveal a tendency towards diabetes (glucose intolerance) that needs to be monitored and sometimes treated like diabetes. Such problems are usually resolved when the corticosteroid dose is reduced or tapered off. Symptoms of high blood sugar include blurred vision, thirst and more frequent urination.

Forgot Your Dose of Corticosteroids?
Take it as soon as you remember (don't wait until the next day). Adjusting corticosteroids without the supervision of your physician is dangerous. If you have to take a lot of medications, you may want to buy a pill organizer that will help you to remember when to take each medication, and will help you to recognize when you've missed a dose.

7. High blood pressure (hypertension): Corticosteroids can increase your blood pressure. If you already have a blood pressure problem, you should watch it closely, particularly when corticosteroids are either started and/or at any time the dose is increased. High blood pressure usually does not produce symptoms, so it's a good idea to monitor your own blood pressure. You can check your blood pressure when you go to the pharmacy, or you can purchase a blood pressure monitor. Note your blood pressure values and show them to your doctor at each appointment. If you do not have a history of high blood pressure, you should still make sure your doctor checks your blood pressure at each appointment.
8. Increased risk of infections: This is due to the effect of corticosteroids on the immune system, particularly when taken in high doses. When you are unwell with fever or other symptoms that suggest infection, seek medical advice promptly. Because corticosteroids can mask a fever, you should call your doctor if you feel persistently unwell even if your temperature remains normal.
9. Swelling or water retention: This is known as edema. People who take corticosteroids may notice that their ankles start to swell. Avoid salty food, and do not add salt to your food.

Long-term Side Effects

Although not all patients experience the following long-term adverse effects, they are common, particularly for persons taking corticosteroids continually for many months or years. Some of these side effects are also related to the cumulative dose of prednisone received (these side effects tend to occur if a greater amount of prednisone has been taken over a given time interval).

1. Osteoporosis: Corticosteroids cause unhealthy changes in bone, known as osteoporosis. People with osteoporosis are at high risk for fractures. Several medications are available to prevent osteoporosis and, in general, one of them should be taken if you are taking 7.5 mg or more of prednisone daily, for 3 months or more (this is discussed in detail in Chapter Six). In addition, it is essential to have a diet high in calcium and supplemented by calcium and vitamin D, as prescribed by your doctor. These preventive measures should be considered as soon as you start on corticosteroids.
2. Glaucoma and cataracts: Corticosteroids may cause the pressure inside the eyes to rise. Untreated and persistently high pressure in the eyes, or glaucoma, can cause painless loss of vision. If you have glaucoma, you should be carefully monitored by your ophthalmologist when corticosteroids are started. If you are taking both an anti-malarial drug and a corticosteroid, it is advisable to have your eye pressure checked. Corticosteroids can also promote cataracts, which are deposits in the lens of the eyes that can cause decreased vision. If these become a significant problem for you, the cataracts can be removed surgically, generally with great success.
3. Avascular necrosis (AVN), also called osteonecrosis: This is damage to your bones caused by impaired blood flow. High doses of corticosteroids predispose people to this condition, although it may also occur in people with SLE not taking corticosteroids. You might experience sudden and persistent pain (often in the hip; sometimes in the knee, ankle, shoulders or other joints). Therefore, you should report persistent, moderate to severe joint pain promptly to your rheumatologist or

Corticosteroids and the Adrenal Glands

Stopping prednisone suddenly when your body has become used to it is very dangerous and could be fatal. Corticosteroids used to treat SLE, such as prednisone, are very similar to the cortisone produced naturally by the body's adrenal glands. These two small glands, located close to the kidneys, produce hormones that regulate water and salt balance, along with many other functions. During corticosteroid treatment, because it notes the presence of prednisone, the body may "turn off" its own production of the hormones that drive the natural production of cortisone. Usually, as the corticosteroid dose is tapered down, the body resumes producing normal levels of these hormones again. However, after a prolonged course of prednisone, your glands may be having some trouble recovering. Some difficulties can occur when the dose of prednisone is tapered below about 7.5 mg per day (since this is comparable to what your adrenal glands would normally produce) if the adrenal glands can't keep up. This is why, if you have persistent fatigue, nausea or lightheadedness as the dose of corticosteroid is tapered down, it is important to inform your doctor; these may be signs that your glands are having some trouble returning to normal.

If you have been taking corticosteroids for a while, and are tapered down to a dose of less than 15 mg of prednisone, difficulty can also occur when you experience some very significant physical stressor, such as an infection or serious injury. In states of severe stress, the body normally produces doses of cortisone that equal at least about 15 mg of prednisone. So, in the presence of significant physical stressors, if your adrenal glands are still on the rebound, your body might not have produced enough natural hormones to maintain the optimal fluid and salt balance. If such a severe stress does occur, it is of paramount importance to inform the doctors treating you for the physical symptoms that you are taking corticosteroids so that they can give you adequate intravenous supplements. Typically, this takes place in a hospital emergency room. You are strongly advised to wear a Medic Alert bracelet. Even if you become unwell and lose consciousness, or if you are in an accident, a doctor will know that you are taking corticosteroids and will make sure that you receive supplements. Very few patients actually run into these problems, but it is good to be aware of their potential, and to discuss your concerns with your doctor.

family doctor. AVN tends to occur symmetrically; that is, if one hip joint is affected, the other hip is prone to react the same. If AVN is diagnosed early, some strategies may help prevent further damage. An example of this is to take the weight off the lower limbs by using crutches, if that is where you're affected. In the worst cases, gradually worsening damage may require joint replacement surgery. In all instances, corticosteroids should be decreased to the lowest dose necessary.

4. Skin changes: If you gain a lot of weight, high dose corticosteroids can lead to permanent reddish or purplish marks (*striae*, similar to pregnancy stretch marks) on your body. Unfortunately, there is not much that you can do to lessen the effects. These marks do fade with time. Corticosteroids may also cause your skin to thin, making the small blood vessels under the skin more noticeable. Changes in the tissues and blood vessels can lead to easy bruising, an effect that usually improves when the dose of corticosteroids is reduced.
5. Heart disease and stroke: In combination with several other risk factors, including SLE itself, long-term corticosteroid treatment can lead to atherosclerosis, a narrowing of the blood vessels of the heart and of the vessels that feed the brain. In turn, this can cause heart attacks (coronary artery disease) and strokes. This may be partly because corticosteroids can contribute to problems with cholesterol. Like smoking, high blood pressure and diabetes, high cholesterol increases the risk for heart disease. As in people without SLE, the risk is lessened when blood pressure, blood sugar and cholesterol levels are well controlled, and when people do not smoke. Therefore, a healthy body weight, a balanced diet, a smoke-free environment and regular exercise will reduce the risk of heart disease. In addition, you may have to take medication to decrease your elevated cholesterol levels.
6. Adrenal insufficiency: If you have been on corticosteroids for a long time, your body might still need dose adjustments at times of physical stress such as during an operation or major illness. You and your doctor need to consider this for up to one year after you have stopped taking corticosteroids. (See the sidebar Corticosteroids and the Adrenal Glands on page 52.)

As SLE gets better, many people logically hope to stop corticosteroids completely. However, it is important to understand that when corticosteroids are used because of severe SLE, the treatment can last many months, or longer. If the dose you take is reduced or discontinued too rapidly, SLE symptoms are likely to recur (that is, flare). Although the aim of both you and your doctor is to reduce gradually the corticosteroid dose as soon as this can be done safely, there is always the potential for flares. Seek medical advice if previously controlled SLE symptoms begin to worsen or reappear as the corticosteroid dose is reduced.

Steroid-Sparing Drugs

There are immunosuppressive drugs that, usually in combination with corticosteroids such as prednisone, are very useful to control severe SLE both on a short-term and a long-term basis. Because these drugs allow people with SLE to limit their dependence on corticosteroids while helping to bring the disease under control and keep it in remission, they have been termed "steroid-sparing." Mycophenolate mofetil, azathioprine, cyclophosphamide and methotrexate are four drugs that can be steroid-sparing.

Why are these drugs given in combination with a corticosteroid drug such as prednisone? Compared to corticosteroids, which start working within hours, steroid-sparing agents are slow acting. They all require at least two weeks to begin their therapeutic action. Patients might see some benefit as early as six to twelve weeks, but significant improvement might not occur for several months.

These immunosuppressive drugs decrease the amount of corticosteroids required to maintain control of SLE, and thus help to minimize corticosteroid side effects. However steroid-sparing drugs do have potentially serious side effects. Good monitoring for the adverse effects can help prevent the toxicity related to these drugs (see page 62).

All steroid-sparing drugs can suppress the bone marrow's ability to manufacture blood cells, which can lead to decreased numbers of red or white blood cells or platelets. Increased susceptibility to infection is also a potentially serious side effect of these drugs, which is further enhanced by their combination with higher doses of prednisone. These infections may be caused by common microbes or by microbes that usually do not cause disease in humans ("opportunistic infections"). When you are treated with one of these drugs, your physician will provide advice on symptoms that could suggest an infection. Such infections always require urgent medical attention because, given the immunosuppressed condition of the patient, they can progress rapidly to threaten's one's life.

All immunosuppressive agents can induce cancers. These cancers are uncommon. All four drugs can cause cancers of the lymphatic system (e.g., lymphomas). As discussed below, cyclophosphamide is also associated with an increased risk for solid tumors such as bladder carcinoma. Because of this risk, your physician will try, whenever possible, to limit the dose and duration of immunosuppressive drug treatment.

Mycophenolate Mofetil

Mycophenolate mofetil (MMF) has been used since the early 1990s for the prevention of acute rejection of transplanted organs such as the kidney or the heart. Since 2000, MMF has gained popularity as a steroid-sparing agent in the treatment of people with lupus nephritis. MMF is taken by mouth usually as a tablet (an oral suspension is also available) and appears to be as effective as intravenous cyclophosphamide in the treatment of major forms of lupus glomerulonephritis (involvement of the kidneys). Although not devoid of potentially serious side effects, MMF is clearly safer than cyclophosphamide in most circumstances. For example, in contrast with cyclophosphamide, MMF is not associated with bleeding from the bladder ("hemorrhagic cystitis") or with infertility due to ovarian failure. For these reasons, MMF is increasingly replacing intravenous cyclophosphamide as the drug of choice for the initial treatment of several forms of lupus nephritis and may allow some patients to avoid cyclophosphamide altogether. Cyclophosphamide, however, is still considered to be the treatment of choice for cases of rapidly progressive lupus nephritis.

MMF is also employed for those who are reluctant to take cyclophosphamide, as a treatment alternative for patients with lupus nephritis for whom cyclophosphamide did not work, or for those who have already suffered cyclophosphamide-associated adverse events that preclude further therapy with that drug (e.g., hemorrhagic cystitis or ovarian dysfunction). MMF is also used as an alternative to azathioprine for maintenance therapy of lupus nephritis, after a 6-month course of cyclophosphamide was successful in inducing a remission.

Diarrhea and a decrease in the white blood cell count are the most commonly observed adverse effects of MMF.

Azathioprine

Azathioprine is a useful immunosuppressive drug that has been used for several decades for the treatment of the more severe manifestations of SLE and for its steroid-sparing properties. However, it is slow to act and has been replaced by intravenous cyclophosphamide and now MMF for the initial treatment of lupus nephritis. Azathioprine is available in tablet form only and the dose varies according to weight. Bone marrow toxicity needs to be closely monitored (see page 62). With such monitoring and dose adjustment as needed, serious blood cell toxicity is uncommon. A potentially serious but rare side effect is liver toxicity, so monitoring liver enzymes is therefore required for this drug. Because azathioprine is often very well-tolerated, it is commonly used over the long-term to maintain remission in previously severe SLE.

Cyclophosphamide

Cyclophosphamide (CYC) is one of the most potent immunosuppressive therapies available. CYC is available in tablet form (given daily), and by intravenous injection (given on an outpatient basis at four-week intervals, often followed by eighweek and twelve-week intervals). Injectable CYC has been used most often over the past two decades for serious SLE manifestations such as nephritis. Although approximately ten times more CYC can be given by injection than by pill, the daily pill format is more immunosuppressive and therefore more associated with side effects such as infections, so it is used much less commonly nowadays. However, oral CYC may still be used in severe SLE, e.g. necrotizing vasculitis (severe involvement of blood vessels causing destruction of tissues). As pointed out above, MMF is increasingly replacing injectable CYC as the preferred treatment for several types of SLE nephritis. However, intravenous CYC remains an important treatment option in SLE when prompt control of the underlying disease is needed, to limit the extent and severity of damage.

CYC can cause hemorrhagic cystitis. To decrease the chance of bladder-related problems, if you are taking CYC (whether daily by mouth or monthly by intravenous injection) you should increase your intake of fluids as recommended by your doctor. It is particularly important to drink fluids before going to bed so that you will wake up during the night to empty your bladder—thereby eliminating the chemicals that may irritate the bladder and cause hemorrhagic cystitis. People taking CYC should be monitored very carefully by their doctors for bone marrow toxicity and, as in the case of all steroid-sparing drugs, regular blood tests (e.g., complete blood counts) should be done throughout the course of therapy.

Nuisance side effects, such as nausea and hair loss, can also occur. This is sometimes seen with azathioprine and methotrexate, but is more common with CYC. Many effective medications are available to deal with nausea, and people receiving intravenous CYC usually receive routinely anti-nausea medications. Hair loss is unpleasant, but fortunately the hair does grow back. You might notice positive effects of the medications also, as the improved control of SLE increases your energy and decreases many other distressing symptoms of active SLE. Keep in mind that, sometimes, steroid-sparing drugs such as CYC may take several months before their beneficial effects are fully appreciated.

Even years after you stop taking it, CYC seems to increase the risk for bladder cancer. Therefore, people taking this drug should have urine tests done at regular intervals for the rest of their lives. Bladder cancer can be treated successfully if caught early. The risk of skin cancer might also be slightly increased when taking immunosuppressives. However, you can minimize other risks for skin cancer: for example, by avoiding sun damage and immediately reporting to your doctor any skin conditions that concern you. Remember that the early identification of these problems will help ensure successful treatment.

Finally, CYC can cause the ovaries to cease production of the normal output of hormones, thereby causing infertility (due to ovarian failure). The risk of ovarian failure related to CYC depends in part on your age at the time the drug is given. The younger you are, the lower the chance of ovarian failure. A sure protection against this side effect has not been completely proven. You should discuss your options with your specialists, particularly if you are a young woman who plans to have a family. If possible, MMF may be considered as an alternative to CYC. The potential side effects of CYC on fertility and pregnancy are also discussed in Chapter Six.

Methotrexate

Certain people with milder SLE manifestations can improve on methotrexate (MTX). A convenient aspect of MTX is that it needs to be taken only one day a week. MTX is considered for people whose SLE causes arthritis or pleuritis (inflammation of the lining of the lungs) that requires frequent use of corticosteroids.

MTX is usually started at 7.5 mg in tablet form and increased as needed to 15 mg per week. When higher doses are needed, or if you have mild but annoying side effects such as nausea, there is a form of the drug which is injectable in the skin ("subcutaneously"). You can learn to inject the MTX yourself. The development of mouth sores and moderate hair loss are possible side effects that are reduced by taking small doses of a vitamin, folic acid.

More serious (although rare) potential adverse effects include low blood cell counts (white cells and platelets in particular) or liver irritation and damage. To monitor for developing problems, your doctor will order regular blood tests (complete blood count and liver enzymes) every two to four weeks when first beginning MTX, and every eight to twelve weeks thereafter. Problems noticed on these tests may lead to a change in dose, or to discontinuation of MTX.

Persistently abnormal liver function tests may lead to a procedure called a liver biopsy. This consists in removing, with a needle, a very small piece of the liver in order to learn if there are any undesirable effects of MTX, or any other liver problems. People with underlying liver disease are usually not good candidates for MTX. Sometimes, you may be asked to undergo a liver biopsy before starting MTX to ensure that this drug will not worsen liver disease that may be hidden on the usual screening tests. It is strongly recommended that those taking MTX avoid drinking alcohol. Discuss this with your doctor.

MTX is usually avoided if you have had kidney damage, because that can lead to increased toxicity from the medication. Hence, monitoring of people on MTX usually includes periodic checks for kidney function.

A rare but potentially serious side effect of MTX is the development of lung inflammation. You might experience symptoms similar to those of pneumonia: shortness of breath, fever and coughing. When it occurs, this complication usually appears fairly shortly after beginning MTX. If you experience this problem, discontinue MTX and seek urgent medical attention.

Also, sexually active women who are of childbearing age should not take methotrexate unless they are on a reliable birth control, because this drug can cause miscarriages and birth defects if taken during a pregnancy.

NSAIDs and COX-II Inhibitors

What They Do

Non-steroidal anti-inflammatory drugs (called NSAIDs for short) can be used either when acetaminophen does not control the pain of SLE arthritis or to decrease chest pain caused by SLE pleuritis (inflammation of the lining of the lungs). There are many different NSAIDs, including aspirin. Some are available over the counter, but you should discuss using them with your doctor because these medications share the same side effects as those available by prescription only. Alternatives to the standard NSAIDs are COX-II inhibitors (or COXIBs), which derive their name from inhibition of the action of an enzyme called cyclo-oxygenase II. Generally you should take only one type of NSAID or COXIB at any given time.

Side Effects

The potential side effects of NSAIDs include stomach irritation or ulcers that can lead to bleeding from the stomach. COX-II inhibitors are less likely to cause ulcers but both COX-II inhibitors and other NSAIDs can affect kidney function. This is a concern, given that SLE commonly affects the kidneys. If you do have any kidney problems, you likely should not take NSAIDs and COX-II inhibitors, so discuss this with your specialists.

These medications can trigger or worsen high blood pressure problems, which should be monitored by you and your doctor. They may also precipitate congestive heart failure in patients with a history of this condition. Another concern is that COX-II inhibitors might increase the risk of a blood clot or other cardiovascular events (heart attacks, for example). In fact, the manufacturer of one COX-II inhibitor (rofecoxib) decided to withdraw their drug because of such concerns. In a review of cardiovascular risk associated with COX-II inhibitors, the American College of Rheumatology did not identify a similar risk for the COX-II inhibitor celecoxib. However, thrombosis has been reported in a few patients with connective tissue diseases (including SLE) shortly after being started on celecoxib. Those patients had antiphospholipid antibodies such as anticardiolipin antibodies or the lupus anticoagulant, which are associated with an increased risk for thrombosis, as discussed on page 33. Because only a few such patients have been reported and because they were inherently at risk for thrombosis, it is unknown whether there was a true cause and effect relationship between celecoxib and thrombosis in these patients.

Patients who are allergic to sulfa drugs (sulfonamides) should not take celecoxib or valdecoxib, as these drugs contain a sulfa moeity. Your rheumatologist will review the potential risks and benefits with you before you begin an NSAID or COXIB. Because the arthritis associated with SLE is often intermittent, people who take them are encouraged to take their NSAIDs only as needed. Also, NSAIDs and corticosteroids can, when combined, increase the risk of stomach bleeding. If stomach irritation is a concern, you can take drugs that decrease acid production by the stomach and prevent ulcers.

How Medications May Be Used in SLE

SLE-related condition	System affected	Examples of treatments
Mild or moderate disease		
SLE-related condition	**System affected**	**Examples of treatments**
Rash	Skin	Topical steroids, antimalarials
Mouth/nose ulcers	Lining of mouth/nose	
Pleuritis (pleural inflammation)	Lung lining (pleura)	NSAIDs/COXIBs*, antimalarials, methotrexate, low-dose corticosteroids
Arthritis	Joints (e.g. hands, elbows, feet, knees)	
Potentially severe disease		
SLE-related condition	**System affected**	**Examples of treatments**
Thrombocytopenia (low platelet count) due to autoantibodies to platelets	Blood platelets	Less severe conditions may be treated with corticosteroids and azathioprine. More severe cases (especially of vasculitis, nephritis, neuropsychiatric SLE and pneumonitis) may require treatments with corticosteroids, mycophenolate mofetil, cyclophosphamide or other drugs.
Anemia due to auto antibodies	Red blood cells	
Vasculitis (blood vessel inflammation)	Skin and any internal organ	
Nephritis (SLE kidney involvement)	Kidneys	
Neuropsychiatric (changes in the nervous system related to SLE)	Brain, spinal, cord, nerves	
Pneumonitis (lung inflammation)	Lungs	

*NSAID = nonsteroidal anti-inflammatory drug (e.g. ibuprofen, naproxen, diclofenac)
COXIB = cyclooxygenase2 inhibitor (e.g. celecoxib, rofecoxib)

Monitoring for Medication Side Effects

Drug	Blood tests	How often	Other tests
Corticosteroids	Glucose, electrolytes (sodium, potassium)	Depends on dose	Blood pressure at each visit
Methotrexate	CBC* Liver enzymes** Creatinine***	Every 8–12 weeks (may be more often in first 3 months or if dose adjustments)	
Azathioprine, Mycophenolate mofetil	CBC Liver enzymes	Every 1–2 weeks with changes in dose and every 1–3 months thereafter	
Cyclophosphamide pills	CBC	Every 1–2 weeks with changes in dose and every 1–3 months thereafter	Urine changes
Cyclophosphamide intravenous injection	CBC	At the time of injection, and 2 weeks after	Urinalysis (as often as the blood work)
Cyclosporine A	Creatinine CBC Potassium levels and liver enzymes occasionally	Every 2 weeks until dose is stable, then monthly	Blood pressure (as often as the blood work)
NSAIDS and COX-II inhibitors	Creatinine CBC	Depends; 2 weeks after starting and thereafter, at each visit.	Blood pressure, liver enzymes and urine analysis

*CBC = complete blood count: includes white cell, red cell (hemoglobin) and platelet counts
**Liver enzymes: markers of liver inflammation
***Creatinine: marker of kidney function (high creatinine means poor kidney function)

FIVE

Complementary Care and Alternative Therapies

Alternative therapies and complementary and alternative medicine (CAM) and care belong to a varied group of systems, practices and products that are not presently considered to be part of conventional (also known as allopathic or western) medicine. Other terms that come up in a discussion of these therapies include unconventional, nonconventional and, more extreme, unproven medicine or health care. There is no or little scientific evidence of the positive effects of CAM therapies. The key concerns of safety, efficacy and side effects are yet to be addressed by submitting these therapies to well-designed, scientific studies.

What Are Alternative Therapies and Complementary Care?

Alternative therapies are a substitute or replacement for conventional medicine, for example, eating a special diet to treat cancer *instead of* undergoing the surgery, radiation or chemotherapy recommended by conventional medical doctors. However, if the diet is used *in conjunction with* the conventional treatments, it would be called **complementary.** Another example of complementary care is massage therapy together with medication to help ease muscle pain.

This chapter will address only complementary therapies. Some examples of specific types of complementary care (that can be combined with your regular medical care) include

- mind-body interventions
- herbs, vitamins and supplements
- manipulative or body-based methods.

Mind-Body Interventions

These are psychological techniques aimed at enhancing the mind's capacity to affect physical function and symptoms. Examples of mind-body interventions include relaxation, (cognitive) behavioral therapies, prayer and meditation, and imagery and biofeedback. These are often taught by specialized psychologists, and can be used to address chronic pain disorders. Some mind-body interventions that were previously considered alternative are now coming to be considered more conventional—for example, patient-support groups and some other types of psychotherapy.

There is evidence that several mind-body therapies, in combination with regular medical therapy, can alleviate the symptoms of disorders not specifically related to SLE, such as headaches, insomnia, chronic low back pain and, possibly, high blood pressure. Recent studies also suggest that some forms of psychotherapies can be helpful for some types of chronic arthritis. However, to date, there have not been many studies of mind-body interventions in SLE specifically. One type of group psychotherapy (brief supportive-expressive) has been studied as an addition to standard medical care in SLE; this study showed no great overall benefit for people with SLE regarding their psychological distress, stress and coping. However, the intervention did decrease illness-related interference with their activities and interests; that is, participants felt better able to participate in activities despite their SLE. Presently, based on this evidence, this type of therapy does not seem to be necessary for all those with SLE. However, if your illness seems to be causing a great deal of interference with your ability to function, you might benefit from group therapy of this or other types.

Other mind-body techniques that can relieve stress and maintain mental health include meditation and prayer. Some studies have suggested that the health of those who partake in activities such as prayer and religious or spiritual involvement has improved. There is increasing interest in how psychosocial factors can directly influence both physiological functioning and health outcomes.

Evidence of the interaction between psychosocial factors and health has been extensively studied in those who have chronic pain syndromes, including chronic back pain, irritable bowel syndrome and fibromyalgia (a non-inflammatory and poorly understood condition with features of diffuse pain and fatigue). If you happen to have chronic pain syndromes in addition to SLE, you might benefit from speaking to a psychologist about the potential benefits of these interventions.

Instructions on meditation can be found in booklets or audiovisual material you can buy at any large bookstore. Your hospital generally will have a chaplain or pastoral care team, who are often very knowledgeable about the role of faith and prayer in illness. They may be able to suggest some reading material, or be able to connect you with other resource people. You may already have some faith practices that you can use to deepen your understanding of your spiritual identity and how your experience of your illness has affected you. Reaching out to family or friends for discussions on these matters may be very helpful. As well, your doctors may know of helpful resources, or be able to refer you to others for additional suggestions.

Herbs, Vitamins and Supplements

Some CAM therapies involve taking substances such as herbs and vitamins. Some examples include dietary supplements, herbal products or remedies, and the use of other so-called "natural" but as yet scientifically unproven therapies.

Use caution when thinking about taking herbal remedies. For example, a study in the early 1990s looked at various preparations of ginseng that had been sold over the counter. It found that some contained several additives that were not listed on the package. Some products contained very little or no ginseng. This lack of purity and a standard are obviously health concerns. Also, severe side effects and even deaths have occurred after the use of some herbal preparations.

One herbal remedy that may have some ability to decrease inflammation and regulate the immune system is the Chinese herbal remedy Tripterygium wilfordii Hook F (TwHF). This has been used for many years in China for the treatment of inflammatory arthritis and autoimmune disease. There is both laboratory and clinical evidence that ingredients in TwHF may have some beneficial immunosuppressive effects in conditions such as rheumatoid arthritis. However, concerns of toxicity must also be addressed. It is difficult to achieve exact dosing of the active ingredient. Also, there are many different formulations available that contain varying amounts of the active ingredient. Additional research is clearly needed to identify the optimally safe and effective dose and formulation.

If you wish to explore therapies such as Chinese medicine, remember that at all times there must be communication between the non-traditional practitioner and your doctor.

Manipulative or Body-Based Methods

Manipulative and body-based CAM techniques are based on the manipulation or movement of one or more parts of the body. Chiropractic treatments, osteopathic manipulation and massage are all body-based methods. There are no randomized trials either completed or underway (as of the time of the preparation of this book) on any of these therapies specifically for people with SLE. However, here are some definitions and some brief notes on some of these methods.

Chiropractic care focuses on the relationship between bodily structure (primarily that of the spine) and function, and how that relationship affects the preservation and restoration of health. Chiropractors generally use manipulative therapy as their main treatment tool.

If you are thinking of consulting a chiropractor (for example, many people consider going to a chiropractor for back or neck pain), talk to your medical doctor first. When visiting a chiropractor, exercise caution, as there are potential risks associated with neck adjustments (including strokes) and some medical doctors feel that they are unsafe. Gentle manipulation for low-back problems may be safe but only if you don't have osteoporosis or fractures in the spine. The careful chiropractor will want to know all about your overall health, all medical conditions and complications (especially osteoporosis or fractures). You should have your rheumatologist's approval before your chiropractor proceeds with manipulations or any other procedures.

Osteopathy emphasizes diseases arising in the musculoskeletal system. It is based on an underlying belief that all of the body's systems work together, and disturbances in one system can affect function elsewhere in the body. **Massage** therapists manipulate muscle and connective tissue to promote relaxation and well-being. **Acupuncture** is an ancient component of traditional Chinese medicine that theorizes that there are over 2,000 acupuncture points on the human body, and that these connect with pathways that conduct energy throughout the body. Acupuncture and massage can be useful for people with fibromyalgia, so if you have this condition in addition to SLE, you can ask your doctor if you can be referred to a therapist.

Although not strictly a manipulative method, **therapeutic touch** is a technique that has some similarities to body-based techniques and some similarities to mind-body interventions. It is derived from an ancient technique called laying-on of hands. It is based on the premise that it is the healing force of the therapist that affects the patient's recovery. There have been a few studies of types of therapeutic touch, but none specifically in those with SLE. As a complementary therapy, it is unlikely to be associated with complications in and of itself. Thus, although your doctor may not be able to recommend this type of therapy specifically, he or she may be open to you combining it with your regular medical therapy.

If You Want to Consider Complementary Therapies

One way to start researching any of these therapies is through your local SLE organization or support group, or, in Canada, through The Arthritis Society. Regardless of the type of therapy or product you are looking into, a few general principles apply.

1. **Talk to your medical doctor.** There may not be much information about the therapy or product you are interested in, as few of these have been stringently tested. Regardless of

that, you need to discuss your plans with your doctor, because even alternative care products have the potential for contra-indications or side effects. For example, some Chinese herbal medicines can cause very serious damage to the liver or kidneys.

2. **Don't give up your regular medications.** Please be on your guard against any practitioner of alternative therapy who suggests that you stop taking your regular medications so you can "cleanse your body" or so that other alternative medications will work. Stopping your regular medication suddenly could cause your SLE to flare badly; *stopping prednisone suddenly when your body has become used to it is also very dangerous, and could be fatal.* If you are unhappy with your current medications, you should discuss your concerns with your doctor. He or she may suggest a compromise: perhaps a supervised trial of a change in your regular medications or the addition of an alternative therapy that is known to be safe.
3. **Be cautious.** Question alternative therapy as you would any other purchase or investment. Those who market a product may believe in it completely, but may not have the necessary medical knowledge about it, nor about your particular medical profile, to be able to assess potential risk. Therefore, do as much of your own research as you can before you make any change in regimen or treatment.

The benefits of many products are "anecdotal"; that is to say, based on an individual's (or many individuals') experience and *not on scientific studies*. The standard way of proving that a therapy is likely to be safe and effective is through controlled research on a large number of people over a specific time frame comparing results with a control group who have not received the treatment. Few types of alternative therapy

Getting Information

Decisions about your health care are important, and you need to be an informed consumer. You should not use a CAM therapy simply because of something you have seen in an advertisement or because someone has told you that it worked for him or her. Questions to ask when evaluating information from an advertisement or site include

1. Who sponsors the advertisement or site? Is it the web site of a manufacturer of the product or drug, or therapy? Or is the advertisement or web site sponsored by the government, a university or a reputable medical or health-related association?
2. With respect to web site information, ask yourself "What is the purpose of the web site?" Is it to educate the public or to sell a product? Then, ask yourself, "What is the basis for the information?" Is it based on scientific evidence with clear references to controlled studies? It may take some thinking to be able to separate out advice and opinions from scientific evidence. (You could try to enlist the help of your doctor in this step.)
3. How current is the information? How often is the site updated?

(Adapted from the National Center for Complementary and Alternative Medicine, Publication No. D167, August 2002, National Institutes of Health Bethesda, Maryland, USA)

have been submitted to such stringent testing. Therefore, be cautious. Also, alternative therapies are not usually covered by supplementary insurance plans and you probably don't want to spend a lot of cash on unproven therapy! Always remember to check with your insurer before beginning a CAM therapy to see if the cost of the services will be covered.

Exercise

Some type of exercise regimen is very important, for several reasons.

- Cardiovascular (aerobic) exercise (brisk walking, bicycling, aquacise, or anything that gets your heart rate up) can limit weight gain and allow better control of diabetes and high blood pressure. This is important because people with SLE may be exposed to corticosteroids that can cause both high sugar levels (and may worsen diabetes) and high blood pressure. These adverse effects may be combatted in part with exercise, which will also hold off the extra weight that also can creep up on people with SLE, either due to corticosteroid exposure or inactivity.

- Exercise improves sleep, mental health and energy levels, and can keep osteoporosis at bay. This is particularly important because people with SLE often complain of poor energy and are prone to osteoporosis.

If you have significant heart or lung trouble, you should talk to your doctor because you may need supervision or help in planning an exercise program. You may need to start slowly, aiming gradually toward the goal of at least thirty minutes of exercise five days a week (or more, if you can). Don't be discouraged if the pace seems slow—keep at it!

If you've been really sick for a significant period of time and your strength or balance is significantly affected, you might benefit from physiotherapy or a supervised exercise

Asking Questions

Here are a few of the questions you should be asking when selecting a practitioner of alternative or complementary therapy, such as naturopathy, homeopathy and Chinese medicine:

1. How much training have you had, and with whom did you study?
2. Are you a member of any professional association; if so, which one, and can you provide contact information?
3. How long have you been practising, and do you have specific experience with SLE?
4. Can you provide references from professional bodies and/or reputable colleagues?

program. People with heart disease also can do very well in a program tailored to them. Ask your doctor about these.

Diet

A balanced diet is important for anyone's general health. Most people have a fair idea of what that means: two moderate servings of protein a day, lots of vegetables and some fruit and some dairy, all accompanied by wise choices of bread or cereal products. If you are watching your weight (recall that corticosteroids, often used by those with SLE, tend to contribute to weight gain), keep portions small, avoid snacking and watch out for calorie-dense foods. People with high blood pressure or problems with leg swelling should avoid foods containing loads of salt (learn to read labels!) and avoid adding salt to your food.

Diabetics and those with impaired kidneys need special dietary instructions. In this case you should be under the care of a specialist, who will provide you with these resources. Also, a heart-smart diet is important if you have high cholesterol or heart problems. Ask your doctor for educational resources and instruction; this may include consulting a dietician.

Vitamins

Few people have enough naturally occurring calcium and vitamin D in their diet. A premenopausal woman normally should take at least 1000 mg of elemental calcium per day. As there is about 300 mg elemental calcium in one serving

Soft Drinks and Osteoporosis

Soft drinks can contribute to osteoporosis. Cola beverages appear to be the major culprits, so pass them up if you can.

of dairy products (a glass of milk or a slice of cheese [about 2 oz, 50 g]), a premenopausal woman needs at least three servings of dairy products per day. Postmenopausal women need at least 1500 mg of elemental calcium a day; people on prednisone also need this much calcium. If you don't like dairy products, or cannot tolerate lactose (a sugar found in milk), you can get some calcium from other dietary sources (almonds, some brands of tofu) but the most efficient way to ensure adequate intake is to take supplements. There are many calcium supplements available. They do not have to be expensive. Check with a pharmacist and double check with your doctor to make sure you are taking the right kind and the right dose.

Vitamin D is present in milk and some other food sources, but taking a daily multivitamin containing at least 400 International Units (IU) of vitamin D will help ensure that your intake is adequate and that your body can use the calcium you take. Persons on prednisone may be prescribed higher doses; again, discuss this with your doctor. There is more information on calcium and vitamin D in the section on osteoporosis prevention beginning on page 91.

Moderate doses of vitamins theoretically could help decrease inflammation, although this is not a well-proven benefit. Such vitamins include vitamin C (500 mg per day), vitamin E (400 mg per day) and possibly beta-carotene. In addition, there is some evidence that alpha-3 omega fatty acids, present in flax seed and in cold-water fish (such as salmon) or fish oil, may be of benefit in chronic inflammatory conditions or if you have high cholesterol. Studies of people with established SLE inflammation of the kidneys (nephritis) proved that taking these vitamins could lead to some lessening of the inflammation, although a long-term benefit was not shown.

Special Diets

Except for the factors already outlined, there is little evidence that either the elimination of certain food groups or a special diet is necessary for people with SLE. However, apart from having SLE, you may feel that you tolerate some foods poorly. For example, as already mentioned, some people are lactose intolerant and/or get cramps or diarrhea from certain dairy products. Less common, but associated with similar symptoms, are allergies to or intolerance of wheat (and barley, rye or oat) products. If you suspect either condition, you can certainly try eliminating the food item in question for a few weeks to see if your symptoms improve, and then discussing the results with your doctor, who might have further suggestions.

SIX

Women—From Puberty to Menopause

SLE affects women more frequently than men; the ratio of women to men with SLE is nine to one. SLE occurs mostly during the childbearing years. In some women, the onset or flares of SLE may be precipitated by pregnancy or by exposure to estrogen, such as when taking oral contraceptives or postmenopausal hormone-replacement therapy. While there is evidence that female hormones influence the functioning of the immune system, their precise role is still under investigation. The current belief is that low-dose estrogen therapy may be acceptable for some women with SLE, although it should always be given under *close medical supervision*. In certain situations, however, exposure to estrogen may have to be avoided. This might be the case, for example, when a woman with SLE has a history of blood clots, or has increased risk of clotting (perhaps due to antiphospholipid antibodies), or if in the past the woman in question had a flare that seemed to be related to a specific estrogen exposure.

The fact that SLE predominantly affects women in their childbearing years strongly suggests that female and male sex hormones (estrogens and androgens) play a major role in SLE. In fact, during all stages of a woman's life, starting with puberty and moving through family planning, pregnancy and menopause, changes in sex hormone levels can alter SLE activity. Conversely, SLE and its treatment can affect a woman's passage through these stages. Thus, this chapter will mainly address how the disease can affect women, and the implications for family planning, although we'll also look at some issues relevant to men with SLE. This chapter is relevant not only to the woman with SLE, but also to her family and friends. There are few things in life more emotionally charged than having children. Therefore, an understanding of and sensitivity to the issues surrounding reproduction are necessary for all members of a "family with SLE."

From Childhood to Adulthood

SLE is relatively uncommon prior to puberty. In North America five to ten cases are found in every 100,000 children. There is only a slight female predominance among these cases. However, at puberty the frequency increases to one case per 1000 to 1500 individuals, with a strong female predominance.

Many physiological changes occur at puberty. In females, estrogen levels rise and the ovaries become functional. Similarly, in males, androgen levels rise and the testicles become functional. The high estrogen state in women contributes to a more reactive immune system. Indeed, throughout reproductive life, the female immune system remains more active than that of a male. After menopause, the immune systems in men and women become more alike, with changes being influenced by fluctuations in levels of estrogen and androgen. Anything that raises the estrogen level tends to make the immune system react more quickly and aggressively, whereas elevations in androgen levels make the immune system less reactive. This concept is important to understand, because it helps to explain the changes in SLE activity throughout life, especially for women.

Ellen had just gone through puberty (at age twelve) when she developed the signs and symptoms of her SLE. Her doctor told her that it was not uncommon for pediatric SLE to occur at puberty. Like anyone her age (or any age!), she found it difficult to deal with the changes that SLE (and the medications that she used) caused. She especially found it hard to go to school or out with friends, when she had obvious signs of the SLE (like facial rashes). Her rheumatologist seemed to understand her feelings, and Ellen felt better knowing that they would be working together to keep the SLE under control. Specifically, Ellen came to understand the benefit of some of the medications she was taking (such as hydroxychloroquine, which greatly helped her rash). She saw that she could take control of her health in many ways (such as by making sure she took her medications properly).

The higher estrogen levels present in women after puberty can make their SLE more active. Subtle changes in disease activity can occur on even a monthly basis. Some women find that just before their menstrual period, they experience increased joint aching and a generalized feeling of being unwell. Fortunately, these symptoms disappear once the menstrual period starts. It's possible that these symptoms indicate a mild increase in SLE activity related to the elevated estrogen that occurs at ovulation. Alternatively, such symptoms may represent a premenstrual syndrome (PMS) that can occur in any woman.

Contraception

Using contraception, specifically birth control pills, is of major importance during the reproductive years. Birth control pills are used not only for contraception but also for regulating irregular menstrual cycles or to relieve severe discomfort during menstrual periods.

Before selecting a particular form of contraception, your doctor will assess your disease, including its activity and severity. Because birth control pills work by increasing estrogen levels, they can aggravate underlying SLE. However, many women with SLE can take birth control pills very well. Nevertheless, monitoring by your rheumatologist is essential prior to and while taking the pill because flares can occur after birth control pills are started. Symptoms of a flare must be reported immediately to your rheumatologist, and the birth control pills should be stopped and avoided in the future.

Sharon, twenty-seven years old, has had SLE for three years. She and her husband have no children, and had hoped to start a family. Sharon knew that she had to discuss this with her doctors, since her rheumatologist had always said that the best chance for a successful pregnancy and a healthy baby was if conception occurred when her SLE was well controlled. Sharon knew also that as well as controlling her disease, her doctors had to carefully review her medications as part of planning the pregnancy.

To be honest, Sharon and her husband were more than a little apprehensive. They knew of women with SLE with kidney damage and other complications related to SLE who were advised not to become pregnant. One of their friends with SLE (whom Sharon had met in an SLE support group) had experienced high blood pressure and a severe SLE flare that had resulted in the premature delivery of her child.

Sharon's rheumatologist had explained that, although pregnancy was sometimes very high risk in women with SLE, in her case, because she had mild SLE and normal kidney function, her chances of a successful pregnancy were good. Sharon was referred to an obstetrician by her rheumatologist, and the obstetrician also thought that Sharon's chances of a successful pregnancy were good. Sharon became pregnant and the pregnancy proceeded well. Sharon's baby was a healthy, full-term delivery.

Here is a list of the criteria and conditions that must be considered when deciding to use birth control pills:

- The rheumatologist will perform a clinical and laboratory assessment to determine the degree of SLE activity when you start birth control pills.
- The disease should be well controlled or in remission.
- Therapy requirements (including low-dose corticosteroids) should be minimal.
- There should be no risk factors for the development of blood clots, such as a previous venous or arterial thrombotic event and/or the presence of anticardiolipin (antiphospholipid) antibodies or the lupus anticoagulant.
- The birth control pills with the lowest estrogen content should be selected.
- Your rheumatologist or family doctor should monitor SLE activity carefully for the duration of birth control pill use.

Fertility and Its Management in SLE

Several studies suggest that there is no difference in fertility in women and men with SLE when compared with the general population. As a general comment this may be correct, but there are exceptions:

1. If the SLE is active and the person with SLE is unwell, problems can occur with women's ovarian function or men's sperm count.

Alternatives to Estrogen-Containing Birth Control Pills

Not all birth control pills contain estrogen. An alternative agent is one containing progestin only. Although these pills have no estrogenic effect and may be safer in a woman with SLE, they may not be as effective as the usual birth control pills, which contain both estrogen and progestin. You can also take an injectable form of progestin, and some find this method particularly convenient. If birth control pills can't be used, the alternatives include condoms (used with spermicidal foam or jelly) or a diaphragm. However, the use of intra-uterine devices (IUDs) is somewhat controversial in women with SLE, owing to an increased risk of pelvic infection.

2. The drugs used to treat SLE can interfere with reproduction. For example, cyclophosphamide can render both men and women sterile, especially if taken orally. There is less risk of sterility if this drug is used intravenously.
3. Some evidence suggests that methotrexate can interfere with the maturation of sperm, but it is not very convincing. However, some physicians recommend that men discontinue methotrexate for three months prior to conception. This recommendation remains controversial, so talk to your doctor.

In cases of infertility not caused by the disease or drugs, the evaluation proceeds along the same lines as for any infertile couple. Medical history and physical examinations are performed, and investigations are undertaken to determine if the woman's fallopian tubes are open and if the man's sperm count is normal. Sex hormone levels are determined for both partners. The cause of the fertility problem can then be treated, if possible.

Often, the treatment of infertility involves placing the woman on fertility drugs. Use of these drugs leads to elevated estrogen levels, which might lead to a flare of SLE. To minimize that risk, the same principles already discussed (the prescribing of oral contraceptives and the planning of a pregnancy) apply to fertility management with drugs. The disease must be under excellent control, with the woman on minimal SLE medication. Flares must be treated quickly and appropriately, and the fertility treatment discontinued.

Becoming Pregnant

In the 1960s, it was thought that pregnancy would put a woman at high risk of a severe disease flare. Fortunately, much has been learned during the past 40 years. With appropriate monitoring and counseling, it has become safer to become pregnant. However, other considerations, such as fatigue, how long you've had SLE and the ongoing, long-term stresses of parenting, must be considered when you are making the decision to have children.

The Pre-Pregnancy Assessment

The woman and her partner must plan a pregnancy in consultation with the rheumatologist. The evaluation prior to a pregnancy involves both a clinical and laboratory review because it is essential that your doctor know your baseline status, so that evaluations during the pregnancy will alert the doctor to an SLE flare. This is especially important if you have any history of major organ disease, such as kidney involvement. Since the normal values for laboratory measurements are different during pregnancy, this baseline is important for the interpretation of later results.

Among the autoantibodies that will be tested for are antibodies called anti-Ro (or anti-SSa) and anti-La (or anti-SSb). These autoantibodies, particularly the anti-Ro antibody, have been associated with heart rhythm disturbances in the babies of mothers carrying this antibody. In addition, the babies may be born with a typical rash (which is described as "neonatal lupus syndrome"). It is important to know the mother's antibody status so that appropriate preparations can be made for the baby at birth. Although this scenario might alarm you, the risk of any problem occurring is only about 3 percent.

The ideal situation for a woman to conceive is when the disease is under very good control, and she is on either minimal or has had no therapy for at least six months. In most of such cases, the pregnancy proceeds well for both mother and baby.

Medication Issues in Pregnancy

The first principle in the management of a pregnancy is that a healthy mother is the first step to a healthy baby. If SLE is under good control, then the rheumatologist will review which medications can be safely withdrawn before pregnancy. Although a woman planning a pregnancy or finding that she is pregnant may wish to stop all of her medications, to do so may endanger both her life and that of the unborn child.

The questions related to medication use during pregnancy are:

- Which drugs can you continue to take during pregnancy?
- Which drugs must you discontinue or avoid during pregnancy?
- Which drugs can you start during a pregnancy should you need treatment for SLE?

Your rheumatologist might suggest the use of certain medications to help you manage your SLE during pregnancy. Comments made regarding any of the drugs are general and may not apply to your specific circumstance. Follow the advice of your own rheumatologist regarding the use of any of these medications. Some are safe in pregnancy; some must be avoided. Be aware that some controversy exists among physicians regarding the use of some medications. Furthermore, a specific drug may be safe for one person but not for another. Each woman should discuss medication issues with her own rheumatologist and follow the advice given.

- Non-steroidal anti-inflammatory drugs (NSAIDs): Among the commonly used drugs in this category are naproxen and ibuprofen. These drugs are usually considered safe in pregnancy up until the end of the second trimester. They should be decreased around twenty-five weeks of pregnancy and discontinued at twenty-eight weeks. These drugs are potentially harmful to the baby close to delivery and therefore must be avoided around that time.
- Antimalarials: These include hydroxychloroquine and chloroquine. Hydroxychloroquine is used more frequently than chloroquine and therefore more is known about its safety in pregnancy. Recent studies have supported the use of hydroxychloroquine in pregnancy. The drug is often continued when a woman becomes pregnant, particularly if there is concern that the SLE may flare if the drug is discontinued. Nevertheless, some rheumatologists are not as comfortable using this drug in pregnancy. Any concern is limited to the first trimester. To avoid exposure during the first trimester, the drug must be discontinued three months prior to a pregnancy and then restarted after twelve weeks of pregnancy.
- Corticosteroids: The risks from taking corticosteroids during pregnancy must be examined from the point of view of both the mother and the developing baby. In the pregnant woman, corticosteroid use is associated with an increased risk of high blood pressure (hypertension) and pregnancy-related diabetes (gestational diabetes). Women on corticosteroids must therefore be monitored

closely so that appropriate treatment can be started as early as possible. The risk to the baby includes premature delivery but this is usually not a major concern because it occurs between thirty-four and thirty-seven weeks, if at all. Recent evidence suggests that there may be an increased risk of the baby developing cleft lip and/or palate. Of course, any potential abnormality causes a parent to be concerned, but this problem is rare, occurring in one in 500 births. This abnormality can generally be readily repaired by plastic surgery. Again, the most important rule is that maintaining the drug is less of a risk to the baby than the risk to the mother, should the corticosteroid be discontinued.

- Most non-steroid immunosuppressive agents should be avoided during pregnancy. The safest one to use, however, is azathioprine. It has a good record in both the mother and the developing baby. Not every rheumatologist is comfortable using azathioprine in pregnancy. Although some controversy exists regarding its use, most evidence supports its use if necessary.

Two drugs definitely to be avoided in pregnancy or at the time of conception are methotrexate and cyclophosphamide. Methotrexate can cause miscarriages and possibly birth defects. Cyclophosphamide is a potent drug with significant risk of causing birth defects in the developing baby. When planning a pregnancy, the woman should be off methotrexate for at least two to three menstrual cycles. At least two menstrual cycles off cyclophosphamide is usually recommended. However, your rheumatologist and obstetrician may advocate longer periods off these drugs before planning a pregnancy, to be more sure that the drug is cleared from your body before the baby is conceived.

Ongoing Management of Pregnancy

Pregnant women with SLE need close medical and obstetrical monitoring. Therefore the rheumatologist and obstetrician must be in continual communication. You will have to have regular visits to both specialists and undergo numerous lab tests. The frequency of these visits and check-ups will depend on your disease activity. When the disease is under good control, and the pregnancy is progressing well, you might be managed by a general obstetrician. If the opposite is true, you will consult an obstetrician specially trained in high-risk pregnancies. Regardless of the obstetrical care, your rheumatologist must remain closely involved.

Flares in pregnancy usually occur in the first trimester (before twelve weeks) and can also be seen within three months after delivery, because hormone levels change during the post-delivery period. Although many physicians are of the opinion that SLE flares are more frequent during pregnancy, this is controversial. Some studies support this observation, while others suggest that there is no difference in the frequency of disease flares of pregnant women compared with non-pregnant women. For many years, it was thought that 70 percent of women experience flares after delivery. Recent studies show that this frequency is closer to 20 percent.

Pregnancy can be particularly problematic for those women who have had major organ involvement, such as kidney disease. They can experience deterioration in kidney function, either due to a flare of the SLE or to the physiological changes occurring in pregnancy. In some cases, the loss of kidney function can be permanent. Such women have to have careful clinical and lab follow-up. Most flares are mild or moderate and can be treated with low or moderate dose corticosteroids, if necessary.

Pre-eclampsia or toxemia of pregnancy may be more common in pregnant women who have SLE. This condition involves high blood pressure, protein in the urine (proteinuria) and fluid in the tissues (edema). This can be more of a problem in those with kidney disease, particularly those who have proteinuria. Your doctor may have difficulty distinguishing a flare of SLE from pre-eclampsia. This is one of the reasons for you to have an accurate clinical and laboratory baseline assessment prior to pregnancy. Again, most flares are mild or moderate and can be treated with low- or medium-dose corticosteroids, if necessary.

Despite advances and improvements in treatment, pregnancy in SLE can be a difficult, occasionally potentially life-threatening, medical and obstetrical challenge. Although with appropriate monitoring and counseling, pregnancy has become safer, women with SLE must be aware that if they choose pregnancy, neither they nor their physicians can guarantee success.

Although there are some genetic links with respect to SLE, it is likely that children of mothers (or fathers) with SLE will not develop the disease.

The Breastfeeding Mother

In general, if a drug can be used in pregnancy, it is safe in breastfeeding. NSAIDs such as naproxen and ibuprofen can be used safely when breastfeeding. The same holds true for corticosteroids, provided the dose does not exceed 40 mg per day. Antimalarials appear to be safe but are a little more controversial. Women have taken azathioprine with little risk to the infant, but cyclophosphamide and methotrexate should be avoided.

Menopause

At the end of her reproductive years, a woman experiences many symptoms due to fluctuating estrogen levels that eventually decrease to pre-puberty levels. These lower levels often result in a reduction in SLE activity. In fact, the female to male ratio of SLE frequency decreases to three to one after menopause.

In the later part of the twentieth century, the symptoms of menopause, as well as other problems experienced by mid-life women, were often treated with hormone replacement therapy (HRT). This meant the women took estrogen orally or by a patch placed on the skin. Many believe HRT has the potential to exacerbate SLE. However, unlike most birth control pills, pregnancy or fertility drugs, HRT provides a fairly weak estrogen exposure and the risk of SLE disease flare is probably not that great. However, recently, studies have shown that users of HRT are at increased risk for breast cancer and other complications. Women with a previous history of breast cancer or with a strong family history of breast cancer should not take HRT.

Estrogen has been commonly used in combination with progesterone, another female hormone. This is because "unopposed estrogen" therapy (estrogen replacement without progesterone) can increase the risk of endometrial cancer (cancer of the uterus). Estrogen replacement can also increase the risk for blood clots (known as deep vein thromboses). By a similar mechanism, it might increase the risk of heart disease. These risks have to be carefully considered if you are considering taking HRT, and should be discussed with your doctors.

Corticosteroid-Induced Osteoporosis

One of the most important concerns for post-menopausal women is osteoporosis. In women with SLE, an additional important risk factor for osteoporosis is whether they have been exposed to corticosteroids.

Marla has had SLE for fifteen years. She went through menopause at age fifty-two. Her family doctor had discussed the options available to her to control her symptoms of menopause and also to prevent menopause-related osteoporosis (bone thinning). Together with her physician, Marla decided that she didn't need medications to control the menopausal symptoms, but agreed that it was important to take adequate calcium and vitamin D to protect her bones. Marla's doctor also suggested that, along with the calcium and vitamin D, she take a medication (called a bisphosphonate) to prevent osteoporosis.

Osteoporosis literally means "porous bones." Sturdy bones weaken, leading to an increased risk of fractures. There are no symptoms until one has a fracture. A woman at age fifty has a 40 percent risk of experiencing a wrist, spine or hip fracture in her lifetime. The strongest risk factors for fracture are low bone mass (as measured by a bone density test) and having previously broken a bone.

Corticosteroid-induced osteoporosis can affect both young and older adults, but typically affects men and women over the age of fifty years. The risk of developing osteoporosis depends upon a number of factors including the dose of corticosteroids prescribed, the duration of use, patient gender and menopausal status. The good news is that corticosteroid-induced osteoporosis can be prevented and possibly reversed.

Corticosteroids and Osteoporosis

Corticosteroid-induced osteoporosis is the most common drug-induced cause of osteoporosis. Significant loss of "trabecular" bone (this is the type of bone found in the spine) occurs with the equivalent of prednisone doses greater than 7.5 mg/day. Individuals who are on this drug for more than three months are at highest risk. The risk of bone loss increases with size of dose and length of time spent using corticosteroids.

What Are Risk Factors for Osteoporosis and Osteoporotic Fractures?

Risk factors for osteoporosis and osteoporotic fractures include both modifiable ones (that you can change) and non-modifiable ones (that you cannot).

Non-modifiable:

- personal history of fracture as an adult
- history of fracture in first-degree relative (for example, mother)
- European ancestry
- advanced age
- female sex
- poor health

Potentially modifiable:

- current cigarette smoker
- low body weight (less than 58 kg/127 lbs)
- estrogen deficiency, including early menopause (before age forty-five), or surgical removal of the ovary
- low-calcium diet
- lack of exercise
- alcoholism

Reprinted with permission from the National Osteoporosis Foundation

The risk of fractures increases in postmenopausal women. Thus, the risk of osteoporosis for a postmenopausal woman with SLE who is on corticosteroids is very high. On average, between 30 and 50 percent of all patients on long-term corticosteroids will experience a fracture if they are not treated for osteoporosis.

Osteoporosis and SLE

There are now several studies showing that bone mass and density is lower than normal in female patients with SLE. Likely, the longer a person has had SLE, the more he or she is at risk for osteoporosis. Corticosteroids play a crucial role in this process, particularly in women (the situation for men with SLE is less clear).

What Is a Bone Mineral Density (BMD) Test?

A bone mineral density test is currently the best way for doctors to diagnose osteoporosis. Your bone mineral density is compared to that of young healthy persons of your sex. Bone mineral density measurements provide the best method for estimating your risk of fracturing or breaking a bone in the future. Measurements are made at several sites; most commonly, at the hip and spine, which are typical fracture sites. The most commonly used bone mineral density test takes approximately five to twenty minutes to complete and is painless, with very low radiation exposure. It exposes you to only one-tenth the radiation of a chest X-ray. On the day of your bone mineral density test, you should wear loose clothing with no metal.

If the test detects low bone density, the results are classified by severity as either osteoporosis, or as a less severe state called osteopenia. Your doctor uses these results to make decisions about therapy to prevent or treat either condition.

When Is a Baseline BMD Necessary?

People receiving any dose of corticosteroids for long periods should have their BMD tested early on in the course of their therapy. A BMD test will help your doctor decide about treatments for preventing and treating osteoporosis. Follow-up BMD studies are recommended for all those on corticosteroids

What Are Symptoms and Signs of a Spine Fracture?

1. Increasing height loss
2. Increased curvature of the spine
3. Sudden back pain (particularly in the mid-back)

Note, however, that only 30 percent of individuals experience pain when they break a bone in their back.

for a year or more. Even with a normal bone mineral density, people can still fracture if they are on a higher dose of corticosteroid for a long period and have other risk factors for fracturing. A baseline X-ray of your mid and lower spine is also recommended if you are on corticosteroids for more than three months.

Jacky is a 45-year-old woman with SLE who was recently diagnosed as having early signs of osteoporosis in her hip and spine. Five years ago, she was prescribed prednisone therapy for three months. She has many of the risk factors for osteoporosis: a family history of the disease; a sedentary lifestyle, as she works at home and does not get much exercise; limited exposure to sunlight; and a diet low in calcium. After reading about the benefits of exercise, Jacky started to do more walking. She was also prescribed calcium and vitamin D supplements, and a medication (called a bisphosphonate) to work against osteoporosis.

Jacky's osteoporosis was caused by several factors: corticosteroid use, SLE itself, her sedentary lifestyle and low sunlight exposure. It is in her best interest to continue walking and to maintain an adequate calcium and vitamin D intake. Since people with SLE generally must avoid exposure to the sun, daily supplementation with at least 400 IU of vitamin D is generally a good idea, although this is particularly important for those on corticosteroids and those past menopause.

Prevention and Treatment of Corticosteroid-Induced Osteoporosis

How Much Vitamin D and Calcium?

A lifelong intake of adequate calcium is necessary for bone health. The combination of calcium and vitamin D can somewhat reduce the risk of fracture of the spine and hip in postmenopausal women. However, calcium and vitamin D are not enough to prevent or treat corticosteroid-induced osteoporosis, particularly if the person with SLE takes corticosteroids for three or more months. In such cases, therapy with a bisphosphonate or other medication is recommended in addition to calcium and vitamin D.

For those taking corticosteroids, total calcium intake from diet and supplements should be about 1500 mg per day. Vitamin D helps your body to absorb calcium. Taking 400 to 500 IU of Vitamin D per day (for persons under sixty-five years) and 800 to 1000 IU per day (for those over sixty-five years of age) is recommended.

The Recommended Daily Nutritional Intake of Calcium (for Persons Not on Corticosteroids)

Age	Intake
7 to 9	700 mg
10 to 12 (boys)	900 mg
10 to 12 (girls)[1]	1200–1400 mg
13 to 16	1200–1400 mg
17 to 18	1200 mg
19 to 49	1000 mg
50+	1000–1500[2] mg

[1]On average, girls go through their adolescent growth spurt two years earlier than boys.
[2]A minimum of 1000 mg is recommended up to menopause in women, with a minimum of 1500 mg thereafter.
(Osteoporosis Society of Canada, Fact Sheet Series Number 3, 1999)

What Foods Contain Calcium?

Calcium Content of Some Foods	**Portion**	**Calcium***
MILK AND MILK PRODUCTS		
Milk—2%, 1%, skim	1 glass[1] (8 oz/250 mL)	300 mg
Buttermilk	1 glass (8 oz/250 mL)	285 mg
Cheese—Mozzarella	1-ounce cube (25 g)	200 mg
Cheese—Cheddar, Edam, Gouda	1 1/2" cube (40 g)	245 mg
Yogurt—plain	1/2 cup (4 oz/125 mL)	295 mg
Milk—powdered dry	1/3 cup (75 mL)	270 mg
Ice cream	1/2 cup (125 mL)	80 mg
Cottage cheese—2%, 1%	1/2 cup (125 mL)	75 mg
FISH AND ALTERNATIVES		
Sardines, with bones	1/2 can	200 mg
Salmon, with bones—canned	1/2 can	240 mg
Fortified soy beverage	1 glass (8 oz/250 mL)	285 mg
Almonds	1/2 cup (4 oz/125 g)	95 mg
Sesame seeds	1/2 cup (4 oz/125 g)	95 mg
Beans—cooked (kidney, lima)	1 cup (8 oz/125 g)	50 mg
Soybeans, cooked	1 cup (8 oz/250 g)	170 mg
Tofu—with calcium sulfate	1/3 cup (3 oz/75 g)	130 mg
BREADS AND CEREALS		
Muffin—bran	1	100 mg
Bread—whole wheat	2 slices	40 mg
FRUITS AND VEGETABLES		
Broccoli—cooked	1/2 cup (4 oz/125 g)	50 mg
Orange	1 medium	50 mg
Banana	1 medium	10 mg
Bok choy	1/2 cup (4 oz/125 g)	75 mg
Figs—dried	10	150 mg

COMBINATION DISHES		
Lasagna	1 cup (8 oz/250 g)	285 mg
homemade soup made with milk, such as cream of chicken, mushroom or celery	1 cup (8 oz/250 mL)	175 mg

*Approximate values.
[1]Calcium-enriched milk—add 100 mg per serving. (Osteoporosis Society of Canada, Fact Sheet Series Number 3, 1999)

Estimating My Daily Dietary Calcium Intake

STEP 1: Estimate calcium intake from dairy products

No. of servings/day		Calcium content per serving, mg	Calcium, mg
Product			
Milk (8 oz)	x	300 =	
Yogurt (8 oz)	x	400 =	
Cheese (1 oz)	x	200 =	

For example, 3 glasses of milk per day provides 900 mg of calcium.

STEP 2: Dairy calcium + 250 mg from non-dairy sources = total dietary calcium

What Types of Calcium Supplements Are Available?

There are different forms of calcium supplements. The preferred forms are calcium carbonate and calcium citrate. Powdered bone (bone meal) or dolomite is not recommended because these have been found to contain high levels of lead. Most of the studies in the prevention and treatment of osteoporosis have used calcium carbonate or calcium citrate.

Since different supplements contain varying amounts of calcium, you may need to check with your doctor or a pharmacist regarding the product you have chosen to ensure that you take the right amount. Some supplements can produce constipation, nausea or upset stomach. Several antacids contain calcium and these can be used as supplements, although this choice should also be discussed with your doctor or a pharmacist. Magnesium supplementation is probably not necessary for adequate calcium absorption.

Lifestyle and Exercise

Cigarette smoking, high alcohol intake and lack of exercise are all modifiable risk factors for osteoporosis. Weight-bearing exercise (for example, walking or jogging) can play an important role in preventing osteoporosis by optimizing bone mass and strength, thereby preventing fractures. Exercise slows bone loss and helps maintain bone mass in people with osteoporosis. Exercise also helps to counteract the effects of corticosteroids, which can weaken the muscles as well as the bones. Back extension exercises can be done to increase the strength of the low back muscles. Posture training exercises may decrease the chance of fractures.

Joan is a 40-year-old woman with SLE who is taking 10 mg of prednisone a day. She takes a multivitamin daily and doesn't smoke or drink alcohol. She has a medical history of blood clots. She has a family history of heart disease and breast cancer. Recently, she developed back pain. Spine X-rays showed a fracture. A bone mineral density test confirmed that her bone mineral density is lower than normal.

What would be the best way to correct or stop this woman's bone density loss? Ideally, it would be best to taper off the corticosteroid if feasible, or reduce it to its lowest possible dose. She needs to have adequate dietary calcium and vitamin D (at least 1500 mg of calcium with 800 IU vitamin D per day) through diet or supplementation. (Note that Joan is currently taking a multivitamin; these usually contain vitamin D 400 IU per tablet.) A bisphosphonate drug is strongly recommended since she has had vertebral fractures and is at increased risk for more fractures. Calcium and vitamin D appear to have positive effects on bone in those receiving corticosteroids, but not enough to be used alone in those individuals taking prednisone 7.5 mg/day or more for three months or longer.

Joan should not take HRT. There is an alternative called Selective Estrogen Receptor Modulators or SERMs. (One example of this type of medication is raloxifene.) These drugs attach to the estrogen receptor, acting differently in different tissues. In bone, they have a positive effect by reducing bone loss, increasing bone mass and reducing spine fractures. Unlike estrogen, SERMs do not stimulate breast tissue and in fact may reduce the risk of breast cancer. SERMs are not believed to increase endometrial cancer risk, therefore progesterone is not required. However, some SERMs may worsen menopausal symptoms, and the risk of deep vein thromboses may be increased, similar to the risk of DVTs after estrogen therapy.

What Other Drug Therapies Are Available for Corticosteroid-Induced Osteoporosis?

Based on currently available information, bisphosphonates appear to be the class of drugs of choice for the prevention and treatment of corticosteroid-induced osteoporosis. If these drugs cannot be used, calcitonin is an effective alternative, particularly in those with back pain secondary to spine fracture. Calcitonin can be administered either as a nasal spray taken at bedtime or as a subcutaneous injection.

How Do Bisphosphonates Work?

This class of drugs works by permanently attaching to bone and reducing the activity of cells that break bone down, thus increasing bone mass. Examples of drugs in this class include etidronate, alendronate and risedronate. These therapies reduce the risk of new spine fractures in patients treated with corticosteroids. Common side effects include abdominal pain and other gastrointestinal symptoms; risedronate may also be associated with high blood pressure and joint pains, and alendronate with heartburn and difficulty swallowing.

Women of childbearing age (that is, premenopausal women) who are sexually active and who are taking bisphosphonates must practice birth control, because exposure of a baby in the womb to these agents could affect the baby's development. Thus, bisphosphonates should be discontinued prior to planning a pregnancy (discuss this with your doctor many months beforehand).

SEVEN

Children and Teens

There are many similarities between adult and pediatric SLE; this chapter emphasizes some differences in clinical features and describes how drugs are used differently in children who have SLE.

Children with SLE complain most frequently about joint pain and swelling (arthritis), fever, lethargy, weight loss and facial rash. The most common serious problem is involvement of the kidneys, which, however, may not cause any symptoms until it is quite serious. This lack of symptoms is an important challenge in getting children to comply with long-term therapy. Children go to the doctor with symptoms such as fever, weight loss and a general unwell feeling with an increased tiredness or fatigue when first diagnosed and when there is a flare of the disease. However, many children and adolescents can have a disease flare, particularly in the kidneys, when they are still feeling well.

Helping Your Child to Understand and Cope with SLE

Chronic, serious diseases such as SLE affect both the body and the emotions. SLE necessitates long-term use of medication, regular doctor visits and other strictures that can be considered, to some degree, "intrusive." They interfere with the living of your child's life. Because of this, both children and adults with SLE can experience a variety of negative feelings that include fear, anger, denial, frustration and depression. It cannot be denied that being either a child or the parent of a child with SLE is not easy. We hope that the following discussion will at least help you sort out and identify some of the possible challenges that you and your child might encounter. We hope also that simply by understanding how and why unpleasant emotions and challenges arise and by realizing that these are not unique to your family, the challenges will be easier to face.

Child Development and SLE

The way children cope with SLE depends on many things, such as the child's age and personality and the severity of the SLE. A child's understanding of health and sickness evolves with age.

Infants and Toddlers (birth to three years) generally have little understanding of their disease. Parents can help by being present for painful events (such as needles or blood draws), and by spending as much time as possible with their child during hospital stays. Parents should interact with their child as much as possible, for example, holding and comforting the child.

Preschool Children (three to five) may understand what it means to get sick, but they don't have a good sense of cause and effect. For example, they might believe that their medications actually cause their SLE symptoms, rather than understanding that they are given to help decrease the symptoms.

Independence is a big issue for preschoolers. Being sick, being in a hospital or being forced to take medications are all challenges to the child's independence. Parents should not be surprised, therefore, to see the child pushing the limits—resisting bedtime, for example. Parents should try to remain firm when necessary, such as when it's time to take medicine. At the same time, a parent can try to offer some choices to the child, and thus help him or her feel a sense of control over their environment. For example, a parent might ask "Do you want to take your medicines with juice or with water?" or "Do you want me to sit beside you on the bed while the nurse gives you the needle, or should I hold you in my lap?"

Early School-aged Children might believe they understand the reasons for their illness, but these reasons may not be entirely logical. For example, they might think they caused the illness by bad behavior. Parents can help by reassuring their child that he or she did not get SLE because it is his or her fault. Make sure the school (and day care staff) have up-to-date information on SLE signs and symptoms. Make sure everyone understands it's not "catchy."

Older School-aged Children are more able to understand their illness and treatment. Parents, friends and teachers who maintain protective barriers must guard against encouraging overdependence in a child. It is not easy for a parent to decide what is excessive or over-protection. If your family is finding this challenging, ask your physician about resources and resource people, for example, social workers and psychologists.

Adolescents begin to develop their own identities and independence from their families. Parents should recognize that it may be difficult to back down from their role as primary caregiver and let the adolescent have more of a role, but these changes are necessary for the young person's emotional maturity. As the adolescent approaches adulthood, the pediatric rheumatologist should prepare the family for a transfer to an adult rheumatologist. Although both the child and parents may experience some anxiety around this transfer, discussions with your pediatric rheumatologist should reassure both the patient and the parents that good care will be made available during this transition period.

Self-image is generally very important during adolescence. That is when changes in the young person's appearance (due to illness or medication) can be a real problem. Also, rapid changes in growth can result in adjustments to medication.

Emotional Impact of SLE on a Young Person

A young person with SLE will likely experience a spectrum of emotions including fear, anger and denial.

Fear and Anger

Fear and anger are unpleasant emotions that are not uncommon in anyone facing illness, including children with SLE. These emotions may arise in a child or a parent when faced with a new diagnosis of SLE, or may develop along the journey as challenges arise. Children with SLE may fear or dislike doctors or hospitals, especially since some of the tests, such as drawing blood or imaging, or treatments can be scary or painful. Hospital stays can be frightening and lonely, too.

Children have as many reasons as adults for being angry that they have SLE. Children with chronic illnesses will feel "different" from other children. They don't want to be sick or to be different. The child's activities might be limited, and sometimes the entire family must change how they live to accommodate this, which can result in feelings of guilt and might contribute to depression. The sporadic nature of the disease is also difficult to deal with. The symptoms of SLE come and go, and children cannot necessarily predict when they will have a flare-up of symptoms—the resulting uncertainty can be very upsetting. Children feel helpless; their bodies are out of control, which can also result in depression.

Denial

Denial is a reaction to an unpleasant situation (such as the reality of having a disease like SLE) that older children and adolescents in particular may use. Adolescents especially want to believe "I'm fine!" even when they feel sick. When a young person with SLE exhibits behavior that suggests she or he is denying the illness, it can be frustrating for other family members, who are trying to be helpful, and for healthcare professionals, who have more difficulty treating the young person if answers to questions about symptoms are evasive or negative. Thus, it may be helpful to have a discussion ahead of time (when the SLE is quiescent) about when and why she or he might feel like denying symptoms.

If you are the parent of a child with SLE, it is possible that you also may have had initial difficulty accepting the diagnosis or that, during a remission, you would like to believe that the disease never existed at all! It is true that the child with SLE should try to lead as normal a life as possible when the disease is in good control or in remission. However, there should be an underlying acceptance that, should the symptoms recur, prompt steps are to be taken; for example, a doctor's appointment is made so that medications will be adjusted to optimize the child's health, so that the child will be feeling well again soon.

Depression

Children and adolescents who have a chronic disease can also become depressed, and it is not difficult to understand why. The stress, symptoms and possible isolation are some important contributing factors. The diagnosis of SLE can turn a family upside down. Limitations may cause depression; for example, if a child is not able to run around and do what she or he used to do. Family members may have to help take more care of them. This can create feelings of dependence that affect the child's self-esteem. Also, if a child is in pain or tired because of the illness, these symptoms can limit his or her activities, which in turn can be upsetting. The child feels different from friends. Sometimes, if the evidence of the disease is visible and obvious to other people, they treat her or him differently, making the child feel embarrassed and inadequate. Discomfort, loss of energy, restriction of activities, disruption of normal life due to medical treatment, isolation from family and friends, and feeling self-conscious, embarrassed or stigmatized can all contribute to feelings of depression.

The early period, when children first begin to understand what SLE is about and what treatments will be used, can be the toughest. This is especially true if the child needs high-dose corticosteroid therapy because of kidney disease or serious SLE involvement with some other body system. This is in part because steroids can cause mood swings. However, changes in appearance associated with steroids also compound the problem, particularly for adolescents, for whom difficulties with self-esteem and self-image can arise.

The other negative effect that medications can have, especially if the treatment regimen is complicated or difficult to follow, is that the young person might have to change his or her lifestyle or need help to follow the treatment regimen. Such lifestyle changes can impose limits on previously enjoyed activities, leading to unhappiness and disappointment. Similarly, overreliance on others for help (for example, by parents reminding adolescents to take medication) might make youngsters feel incapable of doing things on their own, and lower their self-esteem.

As children grow, it is important for them to achieve a sense of independence so that, in adolescence and beyond, they are able to separate from their parents and embark on their own careers and households. Parents of a sick child can seek to protect the child from the outside world, from stress, from embarrassment, etc. This may make sense when the child is seriously ill with SLE; however, when well again, a return to regular activities should be encouraged.

As stated earlier, young people with SLE might at times feel that they are losing contact with their friends. First, they might have less energy or less time to do things like sports and other leisure activities. Second, healthy friends might just assume that certain activities are off limits and therefore not bother to contact friends with SLE. This loss of social contact might also be upsetting and lead to depression.

It is important to help the child with SLE to stay involved with friends, and to find ways to make and maintain new relationships; for example, it might be very helpful for the child to meet other children who are dealing with similar chronic illnesses. Summer camp is a great place to do this. Your pediatric rheumatologist might know of a special camp for children with chronic illnesses, such as SLE, or you should contact your local branch of the SLE association or The Arthritis Society.

Changes in social roles and functioning can arise not just for the child but also for the whole family. Family members might have to take on new tasks, such as driving children to numerous doctor appointments, or feel disappointed if the child can no longer participate in activities that the family used to enjoy together.

Stress, conflict or depression can affect any family member.

Depression is of course harmful because it prevents you from enjoying life and can hurt relationships with family and friends. However, if a child has a chronic disease and also is depressed, the problems can be compounded. For example, the child might neglect a treatment plan and/or schoolwork.

How to Know If a Child Has Depression

Some symptoms of depression in general include

- grumpiness
- irritability or sad mood
- loss of interest in previously enjoyed activities
- strong feelings of guilt, worthlessness or hopelessness

Symptoms and signs of depression can include

- decreased or increased appetite
- weight gain or loss
- difficulty sleeping (insomnia), or sleeping more than usual
- low energy
- difficulty thinking or making decisions

Other signs of depression include outbursts (crying, shouting or complaining) or careless behavior, including alcohol or drug abuse in teenagers. Schoolwork may suffer, and this may be worsened if the child has to miss school because of appointments, or begins cutting classes because school is difficult. Poor communication with (and loss of interest in) people can also occur.

It is sometimes hard to know if a young person with SLE is depressed, as many of these previously mentioned symptoms could be part of the SLE. For example, fatigue and sleeping more could be the result of a flare-up of symptoms, as could feelings of discouragement. Usually these feelings pass as the flare-up passes. However, if a young person with SLE feels sad, down or irritable most of the time and has lost interest in usual activities for several (more than two) weeks, you should also consider the possibility your child is depressed. This is particularly true if some of the other symptoms listed on page 105 are also present.

Managing and Treating Depression

It is important that parents talk to their child about how she or he is feeling. Such communication will help parents develop a better understanding of what their child is experiencing and how to help. At the same time, parents can try to minimize or prevent the child's withdrawal from family and friends—to help the child reach out to them—and, if necessary, adjust participation in activities.

As well, when you suspect depression, inform the young person's doctor. Together, the family and the healthcare provider can decide what to do. Some strategies could include

- attempts to taper corticosteroids if depression is suspected to be a side effect of the drug,
- enrolling the child or family in a support group, or
- having the child attend individual psychotherapy.

In addition, medication to treat depression might be prescribed. Family therapy, preferably with a mental health specialist who knows about chronic diseases like SLE, might be helpful. The child's doctors should be able to refer you to such help.

Effects on the Whole Family

When a child has a chronic disease such as SLE, the entire family is affected. Parents struggle with their own feelings (including their own sadness, anger and denial) about the situation, while trying to keep up a brave front. Therefore, it is helpful for parents to acknowledge these feelings to each other and to other family members and friends. SLE support groups can also be helpful. It is important to stay hopeful. As much as possible, try not to dwell on negative feelings. At the same time, family members should be allowed to express their fears—it is hard for anyone to feel fear, sadness or confusion and be unable to talk about it!

Because having a child with a chronic illness is stressful and time consuming, it is vital that parents try to make time to be together, for example, in the evening when the children are in bed or during periodic outings, when possible. This allows one-on-one adult interaction that will support their marriage during this difficult time. Similarly, siblings of the ill child may feel left out, and parents need to find a few minutes (even if it's just a quarter of an hour talking while doing dishes together) of

Helping Yourself and Taking Care of Others

As a parent, you need to take good care of not just your children but of yourself and your marriage. Parents with a child with SLE may want to use childcare services or respite care to give themselves a break and to prevent getting burnt out. Speak to your doctor or the SLE association about such resources.

Be available so that *all* of your children can talk about the challenges, difficulties and triumphs they are experiencing. Ask them how it's going, and listen to the answers. Even with these efforts, if you feel that things aren't going as smoothly as you would like, you can ask your doctor about family counseling to help with the adjustment process. The goal of a family should be to try to approach the illness by working together as a team to face new challenges.

As the family adapts to a chronic illness, the needs, limitations and concerns of each individual family member should be recognized, while all aim to continue with "life as usual" as much as possible.

Allow family members and friends to help in any way that they are willing and able. This may mean that extended-family members and adult friends come over for coffee, bring over a meal, arrange playtime with children or babysitting, etc. Friends often wish to help, and just want to know how they can do so.

individual time to focus on each sibling. Parents should remember that these siblings may also experience guilt, jealousy, depression or anger. This is why the siblings benefit from extra attention. It might be helpful to schedule individual time for parents and parent-child "dates," to ensure that there are opportunities for sharing, communication, appreciating the joys of each unique family member and just having some fun!

Communication about Healthcare Issues

Good communication between your family and the school is vital. It will help if parents prepare a list of information for the teacher, principal and school nurse. This is particularly true if the child is undergoing rigorous treatment (for example, with medications that may have adverse effects, such as cyclophosphamide) or if the child has recently been in the hospital. Provide clearly marked instructions for medications. If you have a school nurse, your pharmacist may be able to prepare separate medicine bottles for the school. You need an emergency plan in case the child is unwell at school, and a list of phone numbers for you, your child's care team and other contacts.

If your child has mobility limitations due to SLE arthritis or SLE's effect on other parts of the body, be sure to inform the school team that you need to know about changes in your child's activities, such as gym class, lunch, outdoor recess, etc. You will obviously also have to think carefully about transportation for your child to and from school. Special transport may be necessary, or perhaps you just need to talk with your child's bus driver to explain any limitations or needs that your child may have.

Young People with SLE and Their Peers

Young people with SLE will find that some friendships continue despite their illness. Often, children are remarkably

> **Care Notebook**
> To keep yourself organized, it will help to record all of your child's information in one place. A "care notebook" can be used to keep track of appointments, medications, growth, diet, hospitalizations, immunizations, lab work and test results. Some specific suggestions about how to keep track of all of these details is found at Care Organizing for Children with Special Needs: www.cshcn.org/resources/carentbk.htm. Remember, if you write it down, you don't have to rely on remembering when is the next doctor visit. You should also make a list of any questions that you wish to ask at medical visits. Don't hesitate to call your child's doctor with your questions or concerns.

accepting and compassionate about illness in another child. Unfortunately, childhood teasing is also a reality. Of course, children with chronic illnesses are not the only ones who may be teased. However, a young person with SLE or other chronic health problem may be particularly sensitive to rejection.

Teasing and Rejection

The impact of teasing might be eased by some coping strategies that parents and their child can develop together. Specifically, talk with your child about what she or he might do to solve the problem of teasing. Coping strategies might include encouraging the child to assert him- or herself boldly to the classmates who are teasing, or discussing the problem with a friend or parent. Some children are able to ignore teasing by thinking about other things. For example, if the child on corticosteroids is teased during gym class about being chubby, she or he can resolve that it won't prevent enjoyment of the activity; instead, the child can focus on the sport itself. Schoolwork might be something that keeps kids going at a time when they are not feeling happy about themselves or how they look. The ability to succeed in school can become a great strength. Although long-term studies of how children with SLE fare educationally have not been done, some studies have suggested that children with chronic diseases similar to SLE (such as juvenile arthritis) achieve excellent academic success.

As much as possible, treat the adolescent with SLE in ways that promote a sense of empowerment.

- Plan together the appropriate ways to treat, and live with, SLE.
- Educate significant others. Family members, friends and teachers who do not understand the basics of the disease can be obstacles to living successfully with SLE.
- Provide pamphlets from your local SLE support group to teachers, guidance counselors and even classmates.

It is important to help the teen with SLE feel that she or he can gain control of the disease. Parents must keep in mind also that even with SLE, teenagers are, after all, teenagers. Thus, there should be communication about things all teenagers face, including college planning, sexuality, alcohol and drugs.

Nathan is fourteen and has SLE. His mother is concerned because he missed almost two months of school in the past year, although fortunately he seems able to keep up with the schoolwork. While Nathan seems to have a fair amount of energy during the day, he naps when he comes home from school. Nathan's parents also noted that recently he seems to be moody on occasion.

Nathan's pediatric rheumatologist, Dr. Duncan, discussed these concerns with Nathan and his parents, explaining that the goal of medical treatment was to control Nathan's symptoms so that he was capable of continued participation in school. Dr. Duncan noted that Nathan appeared to be responding to treatment, and he believed the disease would not affect Nathan's school achievement. Dr. Duncan discussed possible reasons for Nathan's moodiness, indicating that he felt it might be the corticosteroids (since this symptom seemed to commence when the corticosteroids began). Dr. Duncan followed Nathan closely and began tapering off the corticosteroids dose as the arthritis and rash improved. Since the corticosteroids dose has been reduced, Nathan's mood swings have mostly disappeared.

Important Signs and Symptoms of SLE

Many of the physical aspects of SLE in young people are similar to those seen in adults with SLE. There are some differences in how these signs and symptoms show up in young people compared with adults.

Skin

The rash of SLE is most frequently seen on the face, and may increase after sun exposure ("photosensitivity", as discussed on pages 35–37). It is important to remember that sun exposure can not only cause the skin rash to increase, but also might actually cause the disease to worsen. When people with SLE have the so-called butterfly rash, they also frequently have a rash on the ears. These rashes will generally heal without scarring. The scarring, circular rash of discoid SLE is not frequently seen in children with SLE. Similarly, although hair loss (alopecia) is common, it is rarely of cosmetic significance. Sores in the mouth are common, although they rarely cause any symptoms. People with SLE can also have small sores in the nose. Sores in the mouth or nose may indicate active disease despite the lack of associated symptoms.

Nine-year-old Jennifer had a persistent fever that her pediatrician thought might be some sort of infection. An infectious disease specialist and a blood specialist saw Jennifer and ruled out infection or a cancer. However, over the weeks, Jennifer's fever continued and she developed a persistent pain in her chest that worsened when she took a deep breath. Her pediatrician ordered several tests, including an antinuclear antibody (ANA) blood test. The result was positive and the family were referred to a pediatric rheumatologist, Dr. Duncan. By this time Jennifer had also developed arthritis and a faint rash on her face. Further tests confirmed the diagnosis of SLE and Jennifer began treatment with plaquenil, naproxen and low-dose corticosteroids. Altogether, it had taken several months from the time of Jennifer's first symptoms to the time when she was diagnosed.

Joints

The arthritis seen in children generally involves many joints, and is usually accompanied by stiffness in the morning. It is frequently quite painful, and can lead to problems walking or doing schoolwork. However, the condition usually responds very easily to therapy, and rarely leads to any long-term disability. Although corticosteroids are a form of treatment for SLE, sometimes corticosteroids themselves can cause damage to a joint (avascular necrosis). Whenever possible, a physiotherapist and occupational therapist should be part of the healthcare team of children with joint problems such as arthritis. Your pediatric rheumatologist will arrange this.

Blood Cells

The blood is involved in almost half of children with SLE. This may include the red cells (which make up hemoglobin, the oxygen-carrying substance in your blood), white cells (which fight infection) and platelets (which help form normal clots after a cut, etc.). SLE antibodies can attack any of these cells, destroying some, thereby interfering with the body's ability to accomplish those important tasks. This type of involvement is also seen in adults with SLE. Most commonly, involvement of this system is detected only through an abnormal laboratory value of a blood test, without the presence of any clinical symptoms.

Low red blood cell count (anemia) can exist without signs or symptoms, although it sometimes causes tiredness and loss of color. In this event, the doctor will suggest medicines as appropriate to combat this aspect of SLE activity, particularly as often there may be other body organs that also need treatment. The treatments can include corticosteroids and other medications, such as azathioprine.

Platelets

Even before the diagnosis of SLE is made, many children develop purple spots on their legs or other parts of their body without having any other problems. This is caused by a decrease of the number of platelets, the part of the blood that prevents bleeding. Low platelet count is called idiopathic thrombocytopenic purpura, or ITP. Interestingly, ITP is the first sign of SLE in 10 to 15 percent of children or adolescents who develop SLE. Although ITP might be the first problem of SLE, most children with ITP do not develop SLE.

White Blood Cells

Usually in SLE, the white blood cell count does not lower to the extent of causing any problems. Your pediatric rheumatologist and other specialists will keep an eye on this, particularly if the child is on medications that can contribute to a low white cell count, such as cyclophosphamide, methotrexate and azathioprine. Your doctors will discuss whether medication changes need to be made, either to combat the SLE effects (for example, by adding corticosteroids) or to combat the medication effects (for example, by decreasing the dose of azathioprine, if that seems to be contributing to low cell counts).

Tom was fifteen when he developed the signs and symptoms of SLE. Like anyone, he found it difficult to deal with the physical and emotional changes associated with the disease, and the medications used to treat SLE. At first, he felt so sick and tired all the time that all he seemed to do was go to school, visit doctors or sleep. But gradually he found his energy returning. When he was feeling well enough, he asked his rheumatologist if it was okay to start going to the gym again. His doctor encouraged Tom to do this, saying that it would be very good for him to get regular exercise, but made some suggestions about starting slowly and pacing himself. Now Tom finds his energy level is much higher.

Brain

The neurological system is involved in many children with SLE. The most common problem is headaches. Headaches can have many causes, including tension, stress or anxiety. However, a headache that is very bad or lasts a long time could indicate a more serious condition, for example, SLE. If you are concerned, speak to your pediatric rheumatologist about the symptoms.

Of particular concern are the school problems that arise as a result of brain or neuropsychiatric SLE. In order to do well in school, children must be able to concentrate. However, when SLE is active, the feeling of being generally unwell or tired (either because of active SLE or sometimes as a result of treatment with corticosteroids) may result in impaired concentration. Because this form of brain SLE is difficult to diagnose, it is important to determine whether poor school performance is a result of the SLE, the stress associated with the disease, stress in the family or because of an unrelated school problem. Therefore, it is vital to identify the reason for poor school performance, because the specific treatment will depend on the underlying causes.

Chest and Heart

Problems with the chest and heart are quite common, frequently showing up at the same time. Both can cause pain in the chest due to swelling or inflammation of the lining of the lungs or the heart. Usually these conditions are easy to treat with non-steroidal anti-inflammatories or small to moderate doses of corticosteroids, although sometimes other medications (azathioprine, for example) are used, particularly if there are other symptoms or signs of SLE that need treatment.

Gut

The most common cause of stomach pains is irritation of the stomach's lining due either to stress or as a result of medications. This can be quite common. More rarely, true ulcers can occur. Both irritation of the stomach lining and ulcers usually are easy to treat. Pain in the lower part of the stomach is most commonly caused by constipation and not SLE. True SLE of the gut is not common, but when it does occur, it can be serious. Usually the person with SLE goes to the doctor because of severe stomach and belly pains or blood in bowel movements. Although very rare, if these symptoms and signs are present, you should seek urgent medical attention.

Dealing with Infections

As already mentioned, the number of white blood cells (which are important in fighting infection) may be reduced or not work well, either as a direct result of the SLE or because of side effects from medications. Consequently, children and adolescents with SLE can get more infections than other children. And they may be more at risk for serious infections. Although coughs and colds are still the most frequent infection seen in children and adolescents with SLE, as parents you should be informed about and aware of the higher risk of serious infection.

When to Call the Doctor

It may not be easy to know when to call a doctor. With time, as parents of a child with SLE come to understand the disease a bit, the decision-making gets easier. Here are a few pointers about some signs and symptoms that, in particular, require prompt medical attention. This is only a partial list; always remember, if you have any concerns, seek medical advice.

- If a child with SLE experiences a new fever that persists for more than one day, seek medical advice immediately.
- Blood in bowel movements or in vomit requires prompt evaluation by a doctor, as it may be a sign of bleeding complications, ulcers or other serious problems. Sometimes blood in the gastrointestinal tract changes to appear black in the vomit or bowel movement, and these changes should also be brought to medical attention. (Note that iron supplements also can turn bowel movements black.)
- Chest pain and shortness of breath are symptoms that should be evaluated by a doctor.

Ask your pediatric rheumatologist early on in the course of the child's SLE which circumstances the family doctor or general pediatrician should be comfortable dealing with, and which require specialist attention. Discuss this also with your family doctor or general pediatrician. Recall that the family, the rheumatologist and other specialists, and the family doctor (or general pediatrician, if this is who provides the most of the general care) are all members of a team. Communication is important, but roles may not always seem as clear as you would like. Ask for clarification if these expectations don't seem clear to all of you.

However, children and adolescents with SLE should not be isolated from other children, unless the other child is seriously ill or has chickenpox. Most viral infections, except for chickenpox, are not particularly worse in people with SLE.

Chickenpox

Chickenpox deserves special attention because it can be a very serious illness in people with SLE, especially if they are on corticosteroids or other immune-suppressing medication such as azathioprine or cyclophosphamide. Fortunately, most children or adolescents will have already had chickenpox or have been vaccinated for chickenpox before they develop SLE. Children and teens with SLE should be checked to make sure they have antibodies against chickenpox, so that their doctors and families are completely sure that the child has had chickenpox. If chickenpox develops or if there has been exposure to chickenpox, the child should be seen immediately by his or her physician, and treated with anti-chickenpox medication. In addition, those who have had chickenpox can develop shingles, in which case, they should also be treated with anti-chickenpox medication.

Immunizations

Another unique challenge for children with SLE is immunization. If the SLE is diagnosed before all the routine childhood immunizations have been finished, the child should complete them. However, if the child is on a high dose of corticosteroids or other immunosuppressive medications (which may interfere with the proper response to the immunization), the immunization might be delayed. In general, the current recommendation is that all children or adolescents with a chronic illness, such as SLE, should receive the flu vaccine each year. There is no evidence that the flu vaccine makes the SLE worse and it appears to help prevent the flu in people with SLE. Discuss other vaccinations (such as immunizations against hepatitis) with your rheumatologist.

Adolescent Problems

In both males and females, the occurrence of SLE in adolescence causes specific problems, in particular with appearance. The facial rash can be particularly worrisome, and as a result may require topical corticosteroids treatment and special makeup.

SLE frequently occurs around the time of puberty. For girls, in addition to the cosmetic problems outlined, there may also be problems with menstruation including irregular or missed periods, or a delay in the beginning of periods. These problems are caused both by the medication and the disease. A loss of menstruation can also be the sign of a disease flare, but regular periods will usually come back when the disease gets under control.

Both SLE and its treatment with corticosteroids can cause growth problems. If at the onset of SLE the young person is still growing there can be a temporary slowing of growth. However, if the corticosteroids can be reduced and the disease controlled, usually there will be catch-up growth. Because SLE can prevent normal growth, if corticosteroids can control the disease, they may actually help growth.

Side Effects of Treatments

Corticosteroids, commonly used to treat SLE, have many cosmetic complications. Specifically, they can lead to more facial hair and pimples and a gain in weight (especially when you are taking high dosages). Although these problems will resolve as the dose is decreased, it may take many months for them to disappear. When a child or adolescent is very unwell, or if it is the first time on high-dose corticosteroids, getting him or her to take the medication is usually not a problem. However, after they have lived through the side effects, it is more difficult to convince them to repeat the medication, especially if they are feeling relatively well. Because the goal of treatment is to treat the disease early (before there is serious damage), many people may begin to feel well early during a disease flare, particularly when the kidneys are involved. In order to overcome such resistance, try to help the child or adolescent understand that early treatment may decrease the total amount of corticosteroids taken, and therefore reduce the side effects.

Prescribing the specific dose of corticosteroids is always a balancing act between its good and bad effects. Because children and adolescents will have to live with SLE for many years and because they may require many courses of treatment with corticosteroids, long-term heart problems can develop. Corticosteroids, in combination with other factors, can lead to early development of narrowing of the arteries as an adult. This also needs to be taken into consideration when corticosteroids are prescribed.

Hydroxychloroquine is also frequently taken by children with SLE. It is a very safe drug with few side effects that seems to control SLE well in many cases. However, one possible side effect is the development of eye problems, including permanent partial visual loss (a very rare occurrence). It is recommended that patients on hydroxychloroquine visit an eye doctor every six to twelve months.

EIGHT

Coping with SLE

Living with SLE can pose many interrelated physical, psychological, social and emotional challenges. A few or many might apply to your experience. You are not alone; others have gone through similar experiences. The good news is that you can learn to manage these challenges successfully.

Here are some strategies to help you cope. They can be used alone or, ideally, in combination. If you have trouble learning these skills on your own, think about seeking professional help from a psychologist or other counselor. Although SLE is a chronic illness, remember that there are things you can do to help yourself feel more empowered and in control of your life. Your doctor or local chapter of the lupus society or foundation can recommend further resources. See also the resources in this book beginning on page 144.

Disease-Related Challenges

Sometimes, it's hard to sort out the specific cause of a symptom. Is it due to the short and/or long-term side effects of treatment? For example, if you have difficulty sleeping, is it because of medications or something else? Careful assessment by your doctor might lead to a change in an existing medication, a new intervention, or another avenue.

Difficult decisions—for example, whether to have children at all, or to delay childbearing—are made all the more complicated by the many unknowns. Although good medical care and self-education are helpful, frequent doctor visits and repeated tests can bring on stress and cause disruption in your life. These negative events or stressors are daily challenges for many people with SLE.

Physical changes in your body, caused by the disease and/or its treatment, can certainly be burdensome to live with. Because of changes in your appearance, you might have difficulties with sexuality and intimate relations. You might experience a decrease in sexual desire. Fatigue or pain can interfere with your ability to function sexually. These are tough topics to discuss with your partner and doctor but need to be addressed.

Some challenges, such as medical procedures, cannot be avoided; some recur, for example, disability leaves from work. Some such as depression can be resolved; others must be accepted.

Psychological Challenges

Some of the psychological symptoms described are temporary. Many are more marked when the disease is active.

Like many people with a severe disease, you may from time to time experience a profound sense of loss: of hopes and plans for the future, of independence, of income and of other losses. Such feelings may, understandably, cause you to feel sad or depressed, and lead to signs of other coping difficulties, such as:

- difficulty in controlling your mood or remaining energized enough to deal with daily stressors
- inability to experience pleasure

- disinterest in friends or activities
- finding the presence of others does not improve your mood
- neglecting personal care
- changes in sleep and eating patterns and sexual drive
- feeling tired continually
- being agitated or easily irritated
- feeling guilty, worthless and/or pessimistic
- frequently having a sense of insecurity about the future
- experiencing difficulty with memory and/or inability to concentrate or make decisions
- crying often
- having suicidal thoughts

Some of these symptoms, such as fatigue or inability to sleep, might be due to the disease and/or its treatment; others might simply be the effect of dealing with the daily burden of SLE. It is helpful to familiarize yourself with the side effects of specific medications and with SLE symptoms so that you will realize when something does not seem directly related to SLE or your treatments. In either case, mention your symptoms to your doctor, so that your physical state and medications can be reassessed in order to rule out any physical cause for your symptoms. Sometimes these emotional symptoms can linger on and intensify. They might begin to interfere with normal functioning and cause problems with work and family. In such instances you may have to consult with a mental health professional to lift your mood and help improve how you function.

SLE patients often grapple with uncertainty. What will happen next? What will these medications do to me? For some, the fact that physicians may not always have the answers comes as a shock. This inability to completely answer your questions arises, in part, because no two SLE patients are exactly alike (hence the subtitle of this book: "The Disease with a Thousand Faces"), and because people experience the disease in a variety of ways. Learning more about SLE can help you feel more in control of your life.

Control is an important issue, especially for people with SLE who, like most people, want to feel they are in charge of their lives even when the disease seems to have robbed them of that option. However, it is important to continue believing that your choices and actions do have an impact on your future. Why is this so important? Because, when faced by stressful events, our reactions are most effective when we believe that those events are not completely out of our control. Remember that better living comes from inside yourself. What you choose to do can make a difference. For example, following a healthy lifestyle, such as exercising regularly and pacing your activities, can improve your symptoms and help you feel more in control.

Elena was a forty-three-year-old woman who had been living with SLE for many years before she sought psychotherapy. Throughout the course of her disease, Elena had incurred many losses, both related to changes in her health and body appearance, and in her roles and relationships. Elena was referred by her rheumatologist to a psychologist for help in improving her coping skills, because some of Elena's persistent symptoms—memory problems, poor concentration, fatigue—seemed to be unrelated to SLE activity, and did not respond to medication changes. Psychotherapy was aimed at helping Elena cope with work demands. She needed to learn how to structure work tasks better, limit interruptions and take breaks. Also, Elena, reluctant by nature to ask for help, was encouraged by the psychologist to use her social support network more effectively.

Two strategies she tried were allowing a friend to help her organize her personal items and visiting other friends when she was having a "good day." She took up yoga as a means to relax and combat her fatigue. At the end of therapy, Elena received a good end-of-year work evaluation and reported being better able to live with the ups and downs of SLE.

Social Challenges

Having SLE affects many of your social roles and relationships. If you are a young parent you might be concerned that you cannot adequately respond to your children's needs. If you are parenting alone you might wonder how to tell a new person in your life about the disease. Often, your family members do not know how to help, especially if you have difficulty requesting or accepting assistance. Sometimes people with family members hesitate to communicate openly about the disease and its impact on them, for fear of hurting one another.

While it is widely known that social support is beneficial to both mental and physical health, people with SLE can withdraw from friends or social activities, due perhaps to fatigue, the inability to plan ahead or difficulty with asking others for support. Also, friends might be eager to provide support when you are first diagnosed or during a flare, but could find it difficult to respond to your needs during the long haul. Sometimes, friends withdraw because *they* have a hard time facing their own fears about diseases and disabilities or they might not know what to say or do to be helpful. Often people with SLE report not wanting to "be a burden" to their family or friends or to seem like they are "constantly complaining." As always in human relationships, communication is generally the key element to overcoming these hurdles. Make a list of what you need and from whom, then communicate these needs clearly to your support network.

School and Work-Related Challenges

Study and work are important parts of life that some people can find hard to manage because of their disease. Problems with memory and attention can make many tasks difficult to perform. Therefore, it might be necessary to take breaks or work shorter hours, which can hinder or prevent you from doing your job. Often, people with SLE worry that stress causes a flare and thus, they restrict their activities too much. Although sometimes your doctor might caution against over-exertion, you should not forget that completing your studies or performing well at work are sources of self-esteem. Discuss your concerns about your school- or work-related goals with your doctor, so that as a team you can work out a plan that will optimize your chances of success without compromising your health. You might find it helpful to talk to your employer about exploring some job modifications such as working flexible hours, working from home or reducing your work hours. If you are at college or university you may find switching from a full-time to a part-time program for a while can lower your stress level.

What Is Coping?

Coping refers to the manner that a person typically uses to deal with a stressful situation. Sometimes, more than one coping response can be effective, depending on the situation and the person. For example, in preparing for a return to work after an SLE flare, a person with a more flexible work schedule might find it helpful to think about ways of changing her current working conditions, whereas someone with a less flexible schedule could use her time away from work to get as much rest as possible before returning to her usual arrangements. Both should consider discussing her situation with her superior or the human resources department.

There is no right or wrong way to cope. Instead, there needs to be a match between the stressor and the coping response to that particular stressor. However, in many instances some coping strategies can protect you, whereas others can make your illness worse. Here are four types of coping that people use to deal with health problems:

- **Distraction:** thoughts or actions aimed at avoiding a preoccupation with the health problem; for example, participate in an unrelated activity, watch a funny movie.

A short-term strategy, but relying exclusively on it is usually not enough.

- **Palliative:** self-help activities that reduce the unpleasantness of a situation; for example, enhance your physical environment, take a soothing bath, listen to music you enjoy.

This coping method is very helpful and can increase your sense of control, especially when there is not much else you can do about the situation, other than wait it out, for example, during an SLE flare.

- **Instrumental:** active, task-oriented behavior aimed at solving problems stemming directly from the illness; for example, learn more about the disease, join an SLE organization or support group, find ways to pace yourself so as not to get too tired.

This coping strategy is effective and empowering in those situations over which we have control (for example, learning to better pace yourself) but less useful in those over which we have little or no control (for example, during an SLE flare).

- **Emotional preoccupation:** focus on the emotional consequences of the health problem; for example, worry about yourself and the disease.

While we all use this strategy to some degree, engaging in emotional preoccupation all the time can be draining physically and emotionally.

Coping Approaches

Here are some approaches that will help support you, regardless of your disease and its attendant levels of activity. Some methods involve changing the way you think, others involve changing how you behave.

Lifestyle

There is no question that whether you are sick or well, a healthy lifestyle is good for your health. What we often question is our ability to change long-standing unhealthy patterns. The first step is to identify what health behaviors you need to change, and take some gradual steps to alter them rather than making drastic changes all at once.

Diet and Exercise

Take responsibility for those aspects of your health that you can control. You can eat a balanced diet, exercise on a regular basis and try to get enough sleep. Exercise has the potential to improve your mood and sleep and increase your energy levels. It might prove crucial in the prevention of osteoporosis and coronary heart disease. If you think that you are too tired or sick to exercise, set yourself some goals that may help you overcome your hesitation. Gradually increase your level of exercise, include activities that you enjoy and schedule a regular time for exercise into every day. Consult your doctor before starting any exercise program.

Smoking

While smoking is a health risk for everyone, it is especially bad for SLE patients who are already at higher risk for heart disease and stroke. Studies have shown that smoking can also worsen your SLE symptoms. Breaking this habit is hard but vital to your health. All addictions are hard to relinquish so, if necessary, get help. There are numerous smoking cessation programs and medications available. Research indicates that it is often helpful to combine medications (for example, the nicotine patch) with advice and counseling when you are seeking to become (and remain) a non-smoker. Again, discuss any such medication first with your doctor.

Stress

Being able to manage stress is helpful under any circumstance. The first steps in stress management are to identify the nature of your personal stressors, and then watch for your physical reactions. In other words, listen to how your body responds. These physical signs are your body's way of telling you to slow down. Some common symptoms of stress include

- headaches
- difficulty sleeping
- fluctuations in appetite
- heart palpitations
- fatigue
- tense muscles, and/or digestive problems

Because some of these symptoms may be due to your illness and/or treatment, it is important to discuss them with your doctor. Once you have identified the factor(s) that may be contributing to your symptoms (for example, when work deadlines loom, pain symptoms seem to increase), you need to find those strategies that will help you cope more effectively.

Strategies that can help you better deal with stress fall into three categories.

1. **Managing your physical responses to stress:** As you probably know, it is difficult to solve a problem with butterflies in your stomach and/or a terrible headache. An important step is to reduce this physical tension. Exercise, meditation and relaxation techniques are excellent methods of releasing tension, and often these elements are combined, such as in yoga or tai chi. Have you ever learned a relaxation technique? If finding a class is difficult, there are audio- and videotapes and DVDs that can help you master a relaxation technique that is right for you. Your doctor, friends and local community resources, such as the library, are further sources of information about specific classes and programs.

Edmond was diagnosed with SLE at age twenty-eight. He had quite severe kidney involvement, which required a lot of medications, and found the 20-pound weight gain and other body changes due to taking prednisone difficult to accept. Initially, Edmond isolated himself from others and was depressed. He was concerned that his illness would prevent him from maintaining his relationships, and especially that he might never have the chance to marry and have his own family. He worried about getting sicker, or even dying. His illness also restricted his ability to work, and he had mixed feelings about moving back home with his parents to save money, in spite of the fact that they seemed anxious to help. Edmond told his doctor that he felt depressed, and they discussed what medication changes might help. In addition, Edmond asked if he should see someone to talk about the personal difficulties he was experiencing. Edmond's doctor referred him to a psychologist, who worked with Edmond to identify the multiple stressors in his daily life that needed to be identified.

In order to deal with these stressors, Edmond learned a meditation technique. He began to be more active socially, despite his negative feelings about his appearance. In sessions with the psychologist, he confronted the reality that illness and death were realities in everyone's life. He realized that it was possible to explore his fears in a way that made him feel empowered and enlightened, and not quite so overwhelmed. Toward the end of psychotherapy, with his mental and physical health improving, he found ways of establishing and maintaining his independence and self-worth. He was successful in reducing his stress and worries (although he still had his bad days!) and had a better understanding of why he feared death. Although he knew that many things about the future remained unsure, he felt that he had learnt very useful ways of dealing with the stresses and uncertainties of dealing with a chronic illness such as SLE.

2. **Changing the way you think about stressful situations:** Many times we are faced with stressors we cannot alter, such as having a chronic illness or losing a job. When faced with these situations, you should try to avoid reinforcing the negative aspects of a situation. Thoughts such as "I'll never feel

A Thought Journal

Situation	Thought	Feeling(s)	Alternative Thoughts
Fatigue at work this afternoon	Oh no, maybe it's the start of a flare. It will be as bad if not worse than before. I'll never be able to perform well at this job. I will lose this job.	Anxiety Fear	I'm thinking the worst again. I feel tired lots of times without it leading to a flare. I have had flares before and not lost my job.

any better" or "I'll never be able to find another job" are often unconscious but are, nonetheless, an extremely powerful influence on mood and the ability to cope. Remember that these negative mantras have been learned and can, therefore, be unlearned. One method of controlling these negative thoughts and images is to keep a thought journal. When you experience an unpleasant feeling, try writing down your situation and feelings. Then, evaluate what evidence you have for talking to yourself this way. Find alternative thoughts that are more realistic.

Take the time to identify and alter your negative thoughts. With enough practice you eventually will not need to write them down anymore. Also, there are some very good self-help books that illustrate this technique in more detail (see Resources).

3. **Change your behavior:** Fatigue, the most common symptom of SLE, can be considered an internal stressor. There are various behavioral means of dealing with being tired. For example:
   - Try pacing yourself.
   - Instead of trying to squeeze everything into "good" days, prioritize your activities by doing the important things first and let go of the less pressing ones.
   - Build in rest periods for not-so-good days.
   - If you can, sleep regular hours.
   - Build pleasure into your life. Take hot baths, have a massage, listen to music, go to a café with a friend.

Does this all sound like just more things to do when you are already overwhelmed? Think of stressful events as money spent and self-care as money saved. Consciously save for unexpected demanding life situations!

Doctor-Patient Relationships

Good relationships with your doctors and other healthcare professionals are a crucial factor in coping with the disease. It is essential that you trust your doctor and feel confident that she or he knows both you and your disease well, and that that one doctor be your primary doctor. This person should keep a copy of all your test and consultation reports so that your care is well coordinated.

If you feel obligated to make sure that you do not take up too much of your doctor's time, this concern will cause stress. You and your problems are worthy of the doctor's time. Research has shown that doctors often fail or simply do not have the time to inquire about or notice their patients' psychological or social problems—so you may have to do it for them.

Finally, patients who are in agreement with the medical advice, treatments, tests and so on that are advised, are more likely to adhere to the prescribed regimes. Therefore, you need to discuss your views and values with those treating you so that your treatment plan is one that you can live with and continue as long as necessary. You should consider your doctor as a source of social support who can provide you with information and help in the form of effective medical care.

Be Prepared

Keep a notebook in which you record all events related to your disease, such as doctor visits, medications prescribed, side effects, procedures done and so on. Then, when you visit healthcare professionals you can accurately report what you have experienced. Write down a list of any questions that you need answered. This is an efficient means of managing the limited time during office visits.

Social Support

Support comes from different sources: family, friends, health professionals, co-workers, groups (for example, churches, clubs, support groups); and fulfils several functions (for example, tangible help, such as doing housework, or emotional help, such as providing a sense of belonging). Research suggests that social supports provide many mental and physical health benefits.

- What can you do to enhance your social support?
- What type of support do you need?
- Should you seek out a support group for SLE?

The answers to these questions depend on your level of satisfaction with your current social support, and on your comfort level with asking for and receiving assistance. Women, in particular, have been socialized to nurture others. Therefore some women find it hard to allow themselves to be nurtured or to say, "Not now, I'm not well enough." You might need to examine whether this is true for you. Optimizing your social support is both part of stress management and a means for coping better. You need to preserve time and energy for meaningful relationships so that they are part of your daily life.

Dealing with Life's Big Questions

"Who am I? Why am I living? What is life worth? Why do people suffer or get sick? Why did I get SLE?" Being diagnosed with an incurable disease prompts these kinds of questions, and makes people consider whom they spend their time with, why they tolerate relationships that are not working for them and what they are doing with their lives. This is a surprising "side effect" of a chronic disease. Although you may not realize any immediate benefit for some time, it can bring changes. It can result in personal growth and the development of positive

Sharing the Load

Clarify how the people in your life can help with your needs. No one person can do it all. Try distributing tasks; for example, ask a neighbor to take your child to school and have your husband cook dinner. Then you and your family may be able to more easily get through the difficult periods of living with SLE.

personality characteristics, such as compassion, that have evolved from your experiences in living with illness.

Acceptance is a turning point. When you refuse to be the victim of SLE and you aim to make the best of a bad situation, you can get on with your life. This may seem like a strange concept to you, because many people are used to considering SLE as the "enemy." However, a struggle against acceptance can take up a lot of energy and leave you little for living well. A shift in your viewpoint might come more readily if you reassess your life goals and adjust them according to your current reality. We all need to have realistic goals that will add meaning to our lives. What are yours? You might keep a private journal to sort out your thoughts and feelings related to some of these questions. Sometimes just writing about trauma provides relief. You do not need to share what you write with anyone. You might not even reread it yourself. It is simply one more way of coping that some find helpful.

NINE

What Does the Future Hold?

Research to discover the cause, and to provide better diagnostics for treatment of SLE, is proceeding at a rapid pace in laboratories and research centers around the world. In a study commissioned a few years ago by Lupus Canada, it was found that there are several hundred active research projects in North America alone. Productive research requires cooperation and collaboration of many investigators in multiple centers. As we try to unravel genetic causes of SLE, the participation of patients and their families is more important than ever before.

People with SLE and their families can be reassured that every hour, every minute, every time their heart beats, someone, somewhere around the world is busy doing research to bring an end to the pain and suffering of this disease. Organizations in many countries are active in supporting and directing SLE research. In Canada, CaNIOS (Canadian Network for Improved Outcome in SLE) is a major research effort to provide important new information to guide diagnosis, treatment and follow-up of people with SLE. Similarly, international investigators from North America, Europe and other continents are combining forces under the umbrella of the Systemic Lupus Erythematosus International Collaborating Clinics (SLICC) research group. At an international level, the International Union of Immunology Specialists and World Health Organization Serology Subcommittee conduct research to establish, monitor and improve standards for the diagnosis of SLE and related conditions.

The Search for a Cause

The search for the cause of SLE has been both rewarding and frustrating. It has been rewarding in that healthcare professionals have gained a better understanding of outcomes in SLE, and in that some advancements have been made in the medical treatment of this complex disease. The sometimes frustrating nature of research in SLE has to do with the fact that this disease is likely due to a combination of factors. There is no single "cause," no single immune abnormality, no single gene or environmental trigger that can be traced thus far to the onset of SLE. However, we do have a wealth of clues that helps us understand the disease more clearly, and we do know how to take appropriate steps to prevent flares and the complications of the disease. These advancements have lead to a greater life expectancy and better quality of life than ever before.

Immune Abnormalities

The cells of the immune system involved in the disease process include lymphocytes, a group of cells that control the immune system and can be directly involved in causing the diseases. One group of lymphocytes, called T-lymphocyte helper cells, provide signals to the body to attack and make antibodies, while another, called T-lymphocyte suppressor cells, directs the immune system to retreat. The signals to attack and to retreat come from chemicals and substances made by the T-lymphocyte cells themselves or from a supporting cast of immune cells. Research has shown that abnormalities in all of these cell compartments can occur in SLE. In a normal situation, the immune system achieves a balance of attack and retreat that depends on the perception of the body that is under threat from a virus, bacteria, cancer cell or other foreign substance. In SLE, the balance is shifted to "attack mode"; the cells responsible for "retreat mode" do not respond adequately, while the cells that make autoantibodies are overactive.

Extensive research has defined many of the signaling chemicals and pathways responsible for these responses. This provides important information about the abnormalities of the immune system in SLE, and also will help to design therapies of the future. These include proteins that target and disable or eliminate the immune cells that make harmful autoantibodies.

Do Autoantibodies Cause Disease?

A question that has perplexed researchers is whether the autoantibodies found in the blood of SLE patients actually cause the disease, or if they are simply markers of the disease and therefore have only diagnostic importance. Research over the past thirty years has shown that antibodies to DNA and a group of proteins known as histones that bind to the DNA can actually initiate and cause progression of kidney disease (glomerulonephritis), a feature of SLE that can significantly affect the quality of life and survival.

It has been shown that antibodies to cardiolipin or phospholipid (which forms an important part of the cell membranes) and proteins that bind to them, can cause blood clots that can lead to stroke, blood clots and spontaneous miscarriage.

There also has been interest in the Ro/SS-A autoantibody because research has shown that it is associated with some unique problems in SLE. For one, patients with this antibody tend to develop sunlight-sensitive skin rashes. In this case, the antibody binds to a deep layer of the skin and causes severe inflammation.

A more unusual association of the Ro/SS-A antibody can occur during pregnancy, and is known as the neonatal lupus syndrome. One main problem that can be seen in about 5 percent of the babies of mothers with these antibodies is a very slow heart rate that appears while the baby is developing in the womb. The Ro/SS-A antibodies can cross the placenta and into the baby's bloodstream, where they may bind to the "electrical wiring system" of the baby's heart; that is, the system that controls the heartbeat. As the baby matures in the uterus, this wiring system can become damaged and the heart slows. Sometimes, the baby needs to be delivered early so that a pacemaker can be installed. Because most pregnant women who carry Ro/SS-A antibodies never have babies with these problems, other factors, including other genetic or immune abnormalities or factors in the environment, may be involved.

Environment

For decades it has been thought that factors in the environment may play a role in the onset of SLE. Possible factors such as viral, bacterial or other infections, as well as drugs, chemical or toxins have been studied.

Some experts wonder if a viral trigger may be a contributing factor in the development of SLE. The hypothesis is that when the virus invades the body, the immune system attacks the virus by making antibodies to it, but that these antibodies resemble a part of the normal human cell. After the virus is eliminated, or goes into hiding, the immune system fails to turn

SLE and Ethnicity

One of the mysteries being clarified by research is the difference in the prevalence of SLE in people of different ethnic backgrounds. For example, in Boston the rate of SLE in African-American women is quadruple that in white women. Research is exploring if pollution or toxic wastes in the form of petroleum distillates are implicated. In a larger context, a multi-center study in the United States known as LUMINA (SLE in MInority Populations: NAture vs. nurture) is studying socio-demographic, clinical, behavioral-psychosocial, immunologic and genetic factors.

off this antibody response and continues to make the antibody that can attack the virus, but unfortunately it also attacks the normal proteins in the body. The search for a single trigger, such as a virus, that might cause SLE has been difficult, and no single virus has been identified as a definite cause.

The list of chemicals and toxins under study includes heavy metals, hair dyes, chemicals used in computer manufacturing (trichlorethylene), silica and other hazards from hard rock mining and other factors. Research in mice has suggested that the problems associated with some heavy metal exposures that cause SLE-like syndromes in animals are due to a specific genetic background. The implications for humans are as yet not completely known. The concern regarding hair dyes does not seem founded, as studies have not clearly shown an increased risk of SLE related to hair dyes. To date, the strongest association of an environmental or occupational risk factor has been shown for silica dust and SLE.

Genetics

Current genetic research on families and twins with SLE has shown that several genes are involved. Technologies developed in the last several years can analyze more than 10,000 genes a day, and hold tremendous promise that within a few years the entire map of gene changes in SLE will be put together.

Once this map is assembled, it will be possible to determine how each individual person with SLE is affected. Then, it might be possible to provide each person with SLE with a tailor-made therapy that addresses his or her specific problem. One of these approaches might take the form of gene therapy. For example, if one or two specific abnormal genes can be identified as controlling the immune-system abnormalities in SLE, it might become possible to replace or change the activity of those one or two genes to cure SLE.

Diagnosis

The diagnosis of SLE can be a challenge to the patient and physician alike. In a typical patient, many months can pass before a diagnosis is reached. Advances in the genetic studies of SLE and in new diagnostic testing will mean faster and more accurate diagnoses in the future.

Advances in Therapy

While improvements in diagnosis are important, a key area of research is aimed at helping patients who currently grapple with the challenges of SLE. Research on new therapies is focused on two main areas:

1. Prevention of complications (such as heart disease, osteoporosis and kidney damage).
2. Development of drugs with fewer and less severe side effects, that is, drugs that selectively target the over-active immune system cells without affecting other parts of the body.

Blood Clotting

Extensive research is now focused on trying to identify high versus low risk among patients with the antibodies that promote clotting (known as anticardiolipin antibodies, antiphospholipid antibodies or lupus anticoagulant). If a highly predictive test for clotting risk were developed, those people at highest risk could receive treatment to prevent the actual occurrence of clots, strokes and related problems.

Nervous System

Advancements in the study of the immune and nervous systems will improve the understanding and treatment of the many forms of neuropsychiatric SLE (NP-SLE). For example, a recent study has shown that anti-DNA autoantibodies may react with brain tissue and cause some NP-SLE manifestations. Studies are currently underway to determine the best form of therapy to counteract SLE antibodies that increase the risk of strokes. New therapies being developed for dementia may also hold some promise for certain people with SLE who have significant impairment in memory or intellect.

Hormone Treatments

Because of the possible link between estrogen and SLE activity, some have wondered if hormone medications with effects opposite to estrogen might benefit people with SLE. A few agents have been considered. One, danazole, has been available for many years, but is not often used because of its common side effects such as facial hair growth.

A hormone-based treatment with fewer, and less damaging, side effects is dehydroepiandrosterone (DHEA), which has been used in a number of trials and could be useful in the treatment of mild SLE. Although this agent is not yet in common use, it might soon become increasingly used.

Combatting Complications

Heart Disease and SLE

It is now generally accepted that people with SLE are at very high risk of developing cardiovascular complications. Coronary heart disease accounts for more than one-third of the deaths in SLE and there is also an increased risk of strokes. Besides SLE itself, some of the risk factors appear to include the use of corticosteroids, smoking and the presence of antibodies that accelerate clotting in the blood vessels. Additional research to understand more completely all the risk factors and ways to reduce them is underway. For example, there are ongoing studies to determine the role of monitoring risk factors in SLE such as cholesterol.

Cancer

There has been a fair amount of research effort aimed at concerns that SLE patients have a higher risk of developing cancer. The information to date is that people with SLE do not have a greatly increased risk of developing cancer over all, except for cancers of the immune cells, in particular, lymphoma. This might be due to the fact that people with SLE have over-active immune systems. Research is in progress to sort out whether medications used to treat SLE play a role. Overall, the chance of an SLE patient getting a cancer is still quite low. The risk of a person with SLE developing a lymphoma after several decades of having SLE is probably less than one in a hundred.

Kidney Diseases

In the past twenty-five years, we have learned much about how the kidney comes under attack in SLE and how kidney damage can be prevented. However, the picture is far from complete, and very few of the genetic and environmental factors that lie behind kidney disease in SLE are understood. Research into specific therapies in SLE nephritis is just starting. In addition, research of the EuroSLE Nephritis Trial and other groups will provide insight into more effective use of drugs, such as azathioprine and cyclophosphamide, that have been available for many years. Other international trials focusing on a newer drug, mycophenolate mofetil, are underway. Research on mechanisms and factors that are involved in kidney disease are still progressing.

Pregnancy

For many years SLE patients were told that they should never become pregnant. However, recent research has shed light on which women are at risk of developing complications. In addition, there is a better understanding of the preventive steps that can be taken to avoid complications (this is discussed in Chapter 6). The presence of antibodies, anticardiolipin antibodies, antiphospholipid antibodies or lupus anticoagulant factors lies behind these problems in some people. Research to unravel the molecules involved in this problem and the reason why these antibodies arise in the first place is underway.

Osteoporosis

Research has shown that people with SLE are at high risk of developing early and rapidly progressive osteoporosis. One of the major factors is the use of corticosteroids. However, other factors are likely involved as well, such as inactivity or the disease itself. Research is also underway to address the most effective ways to prevent osteoporosis and, where possible, to restore bone mass in people who are already affected.

Further Resources

Organizations

U.S.

Lupus Foundation of America, Inc.
2000 L St., N.W., Suite 710
Washington, DC 20036
(202) 349-1155
Fax: (202) 349-1156
www.lupus.org

Canada

Lupus Canada
18 Crown Steel Dr., #209
Markham, ON L3R 9X8
(905) 513-0004
Toll Free: 1-800-661-1468
Fax: (905) 513-9516
www.lupuscanada.org
E-mail: *lupuscanada@bellnet.ca*
For information about local lupus organizations contact Lupus Canada

The Internet

There is a wealth of information and misinformation available online. However, doing your own research is an important part of taking control, so here are a few pointers on evaluating web sites and outrageous promises, in general.

On the whole, common sense is a good guide; always consider your source; and remember that if it sounds too good to be true, it probably is!

If a company or an individual is making money from your use of the service, do not rely only on the information they provide.

In general, a good place to start on the Internet research path is with the academic, medical and government web sites as well as associations and institutions.

The following list gives you a starting point:

The ARTHRITIS CANADA web site offers information on lupus and arthritis and on The Arthritis Society, as well as links to other arthritis-related web sites. *www.arthritis.ca*

The Canadian Rheumatology Association web site provides resources such as the CRA Arthritis Handbook at *www.cra-scr.ca*

The Canadian Institutes of Health Research (CIHR) are the major agency funding health research in Canada, including on lupus. Go to *www.cihr-iesc.gc.ca*

MEDLINEplus: *www.medlineplus.gov*

National Institutes of Health (NIH) offers patient education information. To find a list of all the institutes, go to *www.nih.gov*

ClinicalTrials.gov: *www.clinicaltrials.gov*
Canadian Health Network, Complementary and Alternative Health Centre
http://www.canadianhealthnetwork.ca/1alternative_health.html
Contains consumer-oriented, quality assured, web-based resources on a variety of complementary therapies topics.

Canadian Complementary Medical Association (CCMA)
http://www.ccmadoctors.ca/index.htm
Contains links to what the CCMA considers to be the best complementary therapies web sites.

CAM PubMed
http://www.nlm.nih.gov/nccam/camonpubmed.html
Free online searching of the medical literature for information on complementary therapies.

Alternative Medicine
http://www-hsl.mcmaster.ca/tomflem/altmed.html
Canadian site with a great list of links to various sources of alternative medicine information.

WholeHealthMD.com
http://www.wholehealthmd.com/index/
Features the latest news and advancements in complementary and alternative medicine.

HerbMed
http://www.herbmed.org/index.asp
Evidence-based, interactive herbal database. Provides links to scientific data regarding the use of medicinal herbs.

Kidshealth.org contains information on health and illness, aimed at the level of a child.
http://www.kidshealth.org/kid/
It includes a section called "Life with Lupus."

Band-aides and Blackboards web sites for children *http://www.faculty.fairfield.edu/fleitas/contkids.html* and teenagers *http://www.faculty.fairfield.edu/fleitas/contteen.html* with chronic illnesses: Young people can read and share stories about their experiences.

Siblings of Kids with Special Needs
www.med.umich.edu/1libr/yourchild/specneed.htm
Kidshealth.org is a web site where you'll find materials for parents, children, and teenagers on dealing with illness.

Information for the family on dealing with stress can be found at *http://www.humsci.auburn.edu/parent/stress/index.html*

Keeping the family working together when a child is seriously ill
http://www.med.umich.edu/1libr/pa/pa_familytr_hhg.htm

Online Tutorial, X-Plain: Lupus
This online program was developed by the National Institutes of Health and the National Library of Medicine:
www.nlm.nih.gov/medlineplus/tutorials/lupus/id209101.html

Books

Dibner, R., and Colman, C., *Lupus Handbook for Women.* (Fireside, 1994.)

DiGeronimo, T., and Henry, S., *New Hope for People with Lupus.* (Prima Lifestyles, 2002.)

Phillips, Robert, *Coping with Lupus: A Practical Guide to Alleviating the Challenges of Systemic Lupus Erythematosus.* (Putnam Publishing, 2001.)

Pitzele, S., *We Are Not Alone: Learning to Live with Chronic Illness.* (Workman, 1986.)

Singer, A., *Coping with Your Child's Chronic Illness*. (Robert D. Reed Publishers, 2001.)

Wallace, Daniel, J., *The Lupus Book: A Guide for Patients and Their Families*. (Oxford University Press, 2000.)

Table of Drug Names

Glucocorticoid	Approximate Equivalent Dose (mg)
Cortisone	25
Hydrocortisone	20
Methylprednisolone	4
Prednisolone	5
Prednisone	5
Triamcinolone	4
Betamethasone	0.6–0.75
Dexamethasone	0.75
Generic Name	**Common Brand Name**
Azathioprine	Imuran
Cyclophosphamide	Procytox Cytoxan
Mycophenolate mofetil	CellCept
Hydroxychloroquine	Plaquenil
Chloroquine	Aralen
Methotrexate	Rheumatrex
Cyclosporine A	Neoral
Etidronate	Didronel
Alendronate	Fosamax
Risedronate	Actonel

Glossary

Acute cutaneous lupus erythematosus (ACLE): a type of rash that generally involves sun-exposed skin, particularly of the face. When it involves the face, this type of rash is also known as the "butterfly" or "malar" rash of SLE (see "Malar rash").

ANA test: antinuclear autoantibody blood test, done as part of the medical work-up to diagnose SLE.

Antiphospholipid syndrome: a condition associated with specific antibodies (called "antiphospholipid"or "anticardiolipin" antibodies, or the "lupus anticoagulant") that can lead to abnormal blood clotting or recurrent pregnancy losses.

Arthritis: painful swelling of one or several joints. Redness and heat may be present as well.

Aseptic meningitis: inflammation of part of the central nervous system (the "meninges"), which is associated with severe headache and neck stiffness, similar to that seen in bacterial or viral meningitis, but caused instead by SLE.

Autoimmune disease: disease in which the body's immune system attacks itself. SLE is an autoimmune disease.

Avascular necrosis (AVN), also called osteonecrosis: damage to bone caused by impaired blood flow.

Biopsy: removal of a small piece of tissue from an affected organ as part of the process of diagnosing a disease.

Bone mineral density (BMD) test: a test used to diagnose osteoporosis and osteopenia (see "Osteoporosis").

Cataracts: deposits in the lens of the eyes. These deposits can cause decreased vision.

Central nervous system: the brain and spinal cord.

Chorea: involuntary tremor or movement.

Chronic cutaneous lupus erythematosus (CCLE): a skin condition that can be separate from SLE (systemic lupus erythematosus). CCLE can also be a feature of SLE. The typical lesion of CCLE is called discoid lupus erythematosus (DLE); "discoid" refers to the appearance of red, raised, scaly and disc-like patches.

Chronic disease: one that lasts for a long time or for the rest of a person's life.

Cognitive dysfunction: problems with memory and thought.

Cranial neuropathies: nerve problems related to the head and face.

Creatinine: chemical produced by the muscles and cleared through the kidneys.

Dermatologist: doctor specializing in skin disease.

Discoid rash: red, raised, scaling patches anywhere on the body.

Fibromyalgia (FM): condition in which people have chronic, widespread muscle pain and tenderness. Fatigue is also common.

Flare: period when a disease is active, producing symptoms.

Glaucoma: high pressure in the eyes that can lead to blindness.

Glomeruli: tiny filters in the kidneys that filter the blood and allow water, waste (urea, creatinine) and minerals (sodium, potassium, calcium and phosphorus) to pass through the tubes or "tubules" and out into the blood or bladder.

Guillain-Barré Syndrome: rapidly progressing weakness, generally of the legs, that usually is gradually reversible.

Hematological: pertaining to the blood.

Hematologist: doctor specializing in disorders of the blood cells.

Hematuria: blood present in the urine that indicates the glomeruli are not working properly (see "Glomeruli").

Hypertension: high blood pressure.

Idiopathic thrombocytopenic purpura (ITP): purple spots on the legs or other parts of the body caused by a decrease of the number of platelets, the part of the blood that prevents bleeding.

Immune system: the system that protects you from foreign organisms, such as bacteria, viruses and parasites, invading your body. The system is composed of white blood cells (including T and B lymphocytes) and antibodies (made by the activation of these cells).

Immunologist: doctor specializing in allergies and the immune system.

Lymphocytes: B and T lymphocytes are special types of white cells. Some B cells become "plasma cells," which produce antibodies to fight off infection. Sometimes, these antibodies target normal tissue, causing "autoimmune disease" (see "Autoimmune disease").

Magnetic resonance imaging (MRI): a diagnostic technique that uses a magnetic field to produce an image.

Malar rash: fixed red rash over the cheeks (also known as the "butterfly" rash). This rash is symmetric—on both sides of the face—with redness (erythema) and swelling (edema) of the skin over the nose and cheeks (see also "Acute cutaneous lupus erythematosus").

Mononeuritis multiplex: non-symmetrical nerve involvement, causing loss of power or sensation in one or several parts of the body.

Nephrologist: doctor specializing in kidney disease.

Non-steroidal anti-inflammatory drugs (NSAIDs): drugs that decrease inflammation and can be used to control pain, such as naproxen and ibuprofen. They can lead to changes in kidney function or blood pressure, and may also cause stomach ulcers. Thus, the use of these drugs should be supervised by a physician.

Osteoporosis: literally "porous bones," a condition caused by insufficient calcium in the bones from dietary causes, disease, aging or as a side effect from taking corticosteroids or other medications. Osteoporosis causes bones to become more fragile and susceptible to fracture. Osteopenia is a related condition, where the bone changes are not as advanced. Both osteoporosis and osteopenia may be treated with calcium and vitamin D supplements, as well as with other drugs.

Peripheral nervous system: the nerves in the arms and legs that control movement and provide sensation.

Photosensitivity: skin sensitivity in which a rash develops after exposure to the sun.

Proteinuria: protein present in the urea that indicates the glomeruli are not working properly (see "Glomeruli").

Psychosis: distorted perceptions of reality.

Remission: a period when a disease does not appear to be active or producing symptoms.

Renal: pertaining to the kidneys.

Rheumatologist: doctor specializing in lupus and other types of arthritis (of which there are over 100 causes).

Sensory-motor neuropathy: Problems with the peripheral nervous system (see "peripheral nervous system") that can cause problems with movement or sensation, which occurs in a symmetrical manner.

Serositis: inflammation of a lining around a body organ, such as the lungs ("pleuritis"), or the heart ("pericarditis") .

SLE glomerulonephritis, or nephritis: inflammation of the kidneys, a potentially serious but usually treatable condition in SLE.

Sulfonamides (Sulfa drugs): drugs that are best avoided in SLE because they often cause a toxic reation similar to a lupus flare (see pages 3 and 61).

Systemic lupus erythematosus (SLE): a chronic disease with a variety of symptoms caused by inflammation in one or more parts of the body. Often considered to belong to the same family of diseases that includes rheumatoid arthritis, scleroderma and other "autoimmune" conditions (see "Autoimmune disease"), SLE can target any of the body's tissues, including the skin and kidneys.

Thrombotic event: formation of a blood clot in a vein or an artery.

Transverse myelopathy: spinal cord inflammation or damage.

Vasculitis: inflammation of a blood vessel wall, causing a reduction of blood flow.

Index

Note: A page number in italic indicates a figure, table or sidebar.